THE HEART BRAIN
REVOLUTION

The Heart Brain Revolution

THE SCIENCE OF
BEING HUMAN

Ana Maria Stoica

Ana Maria Stoica

Contents

I gather pieces of me
From all of the places,
From all of the times,
From all of the well-hidden memories.
And with each piece I put back
I'm bewildered at the feeling it carried,
A feeling of being "me" that seems so familiar,
And yet, I didn't even know that it was missing!
I didn't even know that I was missing it,
Until I rescued it from being stuck
In that same place, in that same time, in that unconscious frozen
cage.
I didn't know I lost so many parts of me,
Until I got them back.

"REUNION" – ANA MARIA STOICA

PREFACE

This book separates the emotional from the mental.

The EMOTIONAL SYSTEM is a SEPARATE, independent nervous system in human biology. Managed by the Intracardiac Nervous System - located in the human heart-, it gets informed by the body, it informs the Central Nervous System, which, in turn, informs the body, and back, in a continuous cycle during our entire lifetime.

We have been approaching the study of Health in the reverse order.

We have an emotional system with its own functioning rules, neurons, pathways, and purpose. We also have emotional health disorders and emotionally induced mental and physical illnesses. Our emotional system is our base system for life. We arrive here with its processes already in place, with instincts, desires, needs. Our entire life as a human is directed by our emotional needs. Life can be only FELT. Machines understand it, but human beings LIVE it through their felt perception of it.

We made HEALTH too complicated because we did not have all the human biology puzzle pieces. Well, now we have another piece in place. Feelings and the Intracardiac Nervous System are related in the same way our Mind is related to the Central Nervous System. It is time to adjust the image and adapt our healing modalities accordingly- unless the purpose is not healing, but prolonging suffering, with a secondary interest in mind. I am really interested, as you should be, too, to notice exactly who is joining this revolution with the hopes of relieving people from illness, and who is fighting against it. The organisations that really want to help people will help improve this discovery, furthering it. The ones who are perfectly content with how things currently are, will dismiss it and try to convince you that it is not true. And yet, YOU KNOW you have emotions. YOU KNOW you have feelings. And you FEEL your pain. **This is your TRUTH.**

INTRODUCTION

The widely recognised definition of the emotional system is that it refers to the psychological and physiological processes involved in the regulation and experience of emotions. It is considered to encompass the neurobiological, cognitive, and behavioural mechanisms that work together to help an individual respond to and cope with emotional stimuli in their environment. It has been noticed that the emotional system plays a key role in shaping an individual's experiences and behaviours, as well as their perception and interpretation of emotional stimuli.

However, no matter how well-put together this definition might sound, in reality, until now, there has been no clear understanding of exactly how the emotional system interacts with other systems in the body, such as the nervous and endocrine systems, to create a complex and dynamic network that helps individuals regulate their emotional responses.

As such, following this gap in knowledge and understanding, and waiting until the scientific research caught up with this need for further scientific proof, the accepted definitions for emotional trauma mix together psychological, emotional and behavioural references, as they are all impacted by emotionally traumatic events. As per specialised literature, emotional trauma is a distressing event or series of events that overwhelm an individual's ability to cope, causing lasting psychological harm. It can result from various types of experiences such as physical, sexual, or emotional abuse, neglect, or severe loss, and can affect a person's thoughts, behaviours, and emotions long after the traumatic event has occurred. Emotional trauma is known to lead to the development of conditions such as post-traumatic stress disorder (PTSD) and other mental health disorders.

Our definition is a little simpler and direct: emotional trauma is damage done to the emotional system.

The reasons for this "emotional damage" are diverse, and some of them are so "small" and normalised in our current society that they are not yet considered as "traumatising." This is due to the lack of understanding of what the emotional system really is comprised of, how it is functioning, and its role.

This is the purpose of this book.

****

The Emotional Integration Therapy mentioned throughout the book is a comprehensive therapeutic approach that makes use of all of the following methods – when needed:

- The Completion Process method – Teal Swan, philosopher, expert in metaphysics, international speaker, best-selling author
- Voice Dialogue method – Hal and Sidra Stone, PhD
- Rational Emotive Behavioural Therapy - Albert Ellis, PhD
- Hypnotherapy – Ibn Sina (Avicenna), philosopher, physician, astronomer, writer
- Somatic Therapy – Peter Levine, PhD
- Meditation method- from the spirituality field
- Deep Breathing method – from the spirituality field

I

DID YOU KNOW THAT THE HEART HAS ITS OWN BRAIN? SCIENTIFIC RESEARCH

The first published reference regarding the Intracardiac Nervous System was by Scarpa in the *Tabulae Nevrologicae* in 1794. Further research was done in the early 20th century by Cannon and Langley, but they still viewed IcNS as "the little brain" of the heart, just a peripheral system receiving its instructions from the brain, entirely under its control.

In 1991, J. Andrew Armour, M.D., Ph.D., was talking in the Journal of Cardiovascular Electrophysiology about intrinsic cardiac neurons, highlighting the need to further analyse and character-ise the complex interactions between these neurons and other intrathoracic neurons, as well as the intrathoracic ganglia and the central nervous system. The focus is still on how the heart brain is entirely controlled and directed by "the main brain".

Scientific questions about the involvement of the heart brain in the regulation and experience of emotions have started to arise with the medical advancement in heart transplant procedures and the first successful heart transplant in 1967. Unexpectedly, recipients of new hearts have come forward with testimonials about having received, along with the new organ, also new emotional tendencies, emotional memories, and new habits!

Dr Paul P. Pearsall, in his book "The Heart's Code: Tapping the Wisdom and Power of Our Heart Energy", draws on a range of scientific research and forwards the idea of "emotional and cellular memory", arguing that the heart has both intelligence and memory, along with the ability to send messages to the brain, thus influencing our thoughts, feelings, and behaviours.

According to case study information gathered by PhD doctors Paul Pearsall, Gary E. Schwartz, and Linda G. Russek and published in the article "Organ transplants and cellular memories" in 2005, the heart transplant recipients testified to have acquired, along with a new heart, also new tastes, likes and dislikes, affinities, behaviours, and even intrusive flashback memories that helped police officers identify the donor's killer (when the donor's death was sudden and highly traumatising).

Following are just a few examples of such cases, analysed and presented to the public:

- A child who received another child's heart approached the donor's mother when she visited his home and tried to comfort her by saying "It's ok, momma!"

- A young man who received a woman painter's heart started loving going to museums and became very physically affectionate with his girlfriend-asking for prolonged cuddles and going shopping together, both activities that he would previously very much dislike.

- An older white man, who used to be quite inclined towards racism, to the point where he initially wanted to refuse the transplant of an African American man's heart in his body, after having received the new organ, not only started inviting his African American co-workers to his house, but he also seemed to feel more at ease with them. In addition, he started to whistle classical music, songs that he had no way of knowing since he had never liked this type of music before. He was told that the donor was taking violin classes and died in an accident, hugging his violin case.

- A woman who got a new heart from a car accident victim reported that every night, when she calmed down and tried to sleep, she felt the impact of the car on her body, through her body, as if it had happened to her.

There are many other testimonials, leading to an increased scientific interest in cellular and emotional memory research. As a result, further modern research has uncovered the existence of a new type of cell in the heart – glial cells.

Scientists used to believe that glial cells are found only in the brain, as their main function is to support neuronal activities. However, they have found a different type of glial cell, with properties similar to those found in the central nervous system, in the pancreas and the lungs, without a clear understanding of their actual function in those organs. Further research discovered a new type of glial cell in the heart – nexus glia, on top of the glial cells they were already aware of being there, that were similar to those in the central nervous system. For example, oligodendrocytes, one type of glial cells, are involved in the production and maintenance of myelin, which is an insulating layer around nerve fibres that helps to improve the conduction of electrical signals- in the brain, as well as in the heart. And, lastly, recent research has also implicated astrocytes in processes such as synaptic plasticity, learning, and memory, which provides a scientific platform for the unexpectedly accurate testimonials of heart transplant recipients- they received their "new" hearts with neuronal cells that had already been imprinted with memories.

WHY IS THIS IMPORTANT?

It is widely known and already agreed that the glial cells found in the central nervous system play a key role in maintaining its microenvironment, being involved in a variety of physiological processes that support and protect the neurons. The ones found in the heart seem to have the same purpose – supporting the good functioning of the cardiac microenvironment and assisting with the proper conduction of electrical signals among intracardiac neurons. And with the glial cells found in the other organs, we can conclude that either there is a mistake in our biology, or there is another type of electrical communication through the entirety of the human body, a "communication pathway" that we have yet to uncover.

On 26th of May 2020, scientists from Thomas Jefferson University published a breakthrough discovery: with the help of a new 3-D imaging technology, they have managed, for the first time in history, to produce a detailed, comprehensive 3-D map of the Intracardiac Nervous System in a male rat heart – **the first 3-D map of the heart's neurons**.

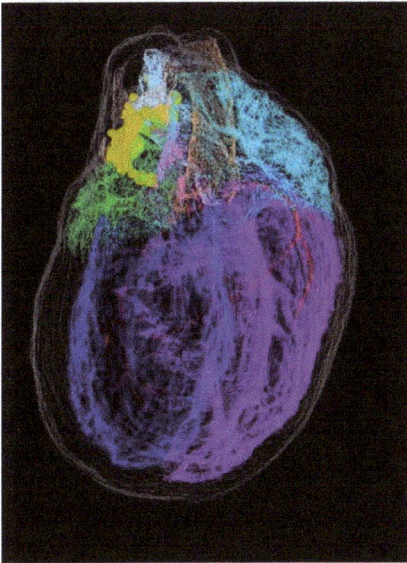

The IcNS is represented by the yellow agglomeration in the top-left part of the image.

The only other organ for which such a high-resolution 3-D map has been deemed necessary, due to the neuronal network complexity, is the brain.

This image shows a whole-heart view of the 3D reconstructed male rat heart, showing the extent and distribution of the intrinsic cardiac neurons
Achanta et al. – iScience

This detailed look at the network of nerves and neurotransmitters that make up the heart's brain has allowed scientists to notice that the intrinsic nervous system within the heart is much more complex and much better organised than expected. They have found that the intracardiac neurons are arranged in a specific and coherent band of clusters, positioned at the top of the heart and extending down, on the back left side of the heart. Also, there is another unexpected observation- **there is a difference between male and female hearts in the way neurons are organised** - both spatially and by their gene expression. This leads the way to further scientific research into the theory that there is a difference in emotional perception between human males and females.

Additionally, new work in the field of neurobiology by Prof. Kokh has recently found that neurons in the main brain give rise to extracellular electrical fields that feed back into themselves and neighbouring neurons, influencing their behaviour. This amazing discovery suggests that the fields may, in fact, represent an additional way of neuronal communication, different from the direct synaptic junctions means of communication known until now. Since IcNS is, in effect, a brain – we can extrapolate that the electrical activity and behaviours that apply to the main brain are, in fact, present in the heart brain, as well – and so, the difference in the neuronal spatial arrangement between male and female hearts is a major factor in the treatment of emotional data, as it decides which neurons are influenced by a specific electrical activity.

Due to this complexity, and the additional scientific findings indicated below, it is safe to conclude that, if up until now, the consensus scientific opinion was that the Intracardiac Nervous System was entirely under the control of our main brain, we can now accept the fact that the heart contains an independent nervous system, with tight connections to the brain, but in an equally significant position, not in a subordinate relationship. Its main function is the receiving, translating, storing, and retrieving of emotional and sensory information, providing instructions to the body and the brain in accordance with the emotional reality it perceives and records.

The connection between the existing scientific findings and the conclusion mentioned above is supported by the fact that we can access early childhood memories directly through the emotional component – the "feeling signature" stored in the intracardiac neurons and the somatic experience – of current events, and that, by modifying the similar emotional component in these early childhood events (emotional integration therapy), there is a clear diminished reactivity when re-experiencing the current ones as an adult.

ADDITIONAL SCIENTIFIC RESEARCH SUPPORT

- Thayer, J. F., & Lane, R. D. (2000). Calm physiology. Psychology Review, 107(1), 71-80)
- Kerr, C. E., & Shaw, J. B. (2017). The heart's role in emotional regulation: A review. Frontiers in Psychology, 8, 1069

These two studies on the anatomy and physiology of the heart discuss the possibility that the heart has its own intrinsic nervous system, consisting of specialised neurons known as intrinsic cardiac neurons. They have also suggested that the heart's neurons may be capable of encoding and retrieving emotional memories, providing a physiological basis for the phenomenon of 'heartfelt memories'. This means that the heart's intrinsic nervous system may **process, store, and retrieve emotional memories independently of the central nervous system, including the brain.** The theory that the heart has the ability to record emotional experiences has important implications for how we approach the notion of "emotional system" and "emotional trauma". Additionally, the heart's neural network has been shown to play a role in regulating emotional responses and behaviours. This suggests that the heart may have a direct influence on the way in which emotional experiences are processed and remembered and that it may play a role in the development of emotional disorders. The study authors propose that targeting the heart's neural network may improve emotional regulation and reduce the impact of emotional disorders, and targeting the interconnections between the heart and the brain may enhance emotional regulation and resilience by improving the processing of emotional information.

- Porges, S. W. (2007). The polyvagal theory: phylogenetic substrates of a social nervous system. International journal of psychophysiology, 65(2), 116-126).

In addition to its role in emotional regulation, the heart's neural network may also play a role in the communication of emotional information between the heart and the brain. This study concluded that **the heart sends a significant amount of information to the brain** through the vagus nerve and that this information is processed by the brain to influence emotional experience. This supports the premise that **the heart serves as a mediator of emotional information between the body and the brain** and that it may play a significant role in shaping emotional experience and memory.

• Armour, J. A., & Ardell, J. L. (2004). Neurocardiology: anatomical and functional principles. Complementary and Alternative Medicine, 4, 14.

Dr. J. Andrew Armour and his colleagues at the University of
Montreal provide support for the conclusion that the heart plays
a role in the perception of emotional stimuli. They found that the
electrical activity generated by the heart can influence the processing of emotional information in the brain, suggesting that the
heart-brain connection plays a significant role in emotional regulation. These findings provide compelling evidence that **the heart
is not just a passive receptor of emotional stimuli, but rather
an active participant** in the emotional experience.

• LeDoux, J. E. (1996). The emotional brain: The mysterious
underpinnings of emotional life. Simon and Schuster.

This study supports the idea that **the amygdala can react before receiving input from the central nervous system (CNS).**
Here, LeDoux proposed a model of emotion processing in which
sensory information is initially processed in the amygdala, allowing for **rapid and automatic emotional responses**, before being
transmitted to higher cortical areas for more detailed processing
and interpretation. This model is sometimes referred to as the
"low road-high road" model, **with the amygdala standing for
the "low road" for rapid, automatic processing of emotional
stimuli.**

LeDoux and colleagues conducted a series of experiments with rats, in which they showed that auditory information could reach the amygdala directly, bypassing the cortex and allowing for rapid emotional responses. They also showed that lesions to the amygdala could impair emotional learning, further supporting the idea that the amygdala plays a critical role in emotional processing.

Further on, there is evidence to suggest that **the heart can send signals to the brain via the vagus nerve**, which is a key component of the parasympathetic nervous system and has connections to the amygdala. For example, research has shown that heart rate variability, which reflects changes in the activity of the autonomic nervous system, is associated with changes in amygdala activation in response to emotional stimuli (e.g., Thayer et al., 2009). Research has shown that sympathetic activation can increase cortisol levels via the activation of the HPA axis (e.g., Epel et al., 2004), while parasympathetic activity can have the opposite effect, reducing cortisol levels (e.g., Thayer et al., 2010). Given that the Intracardiac nervous system is currently considered to be a component of the autonomic nervous system and plays a role in regulating heart rate and other autonomic functions, it is possible that it could also influence hormonal activity via the sympathetic and parasympathetic pathways.

- Thayer, J. F., & Lane, R. D. (2009). Claude Bernard and the heart-brain connection: further elaboration of a model of neurovisceral integration. Neuropsychologia, 47(10), 2064-2068.
- Chittka, L., & Niven, J. (2009). Are bigger brains better? Curr Biol, 19(19), R995-1008.

• McCraty, R., Barrios-Choplin, B., Rozman, D., Atkinson, M., & Watkins, A. D. (1998). The Coherent Heart: Heart-Brain Interactions, Psychophysiological Coherence, and the Emergence of System-Wide Order. Integrative Physiological & Behavioural Science, 33(2), 151–170.

From these studies, we can conclude that **the heart can respond to emotionally charged events**, with changes in heart rate and rhythm being recorded. In addition, they have also suggested that **the heart's neural activity may be capable of recording emotional memory**, which has significant implications for our understanding of the emotional experience. Additionally, it was found that participants who viewed emotionally charged images exhibited changes in heart rate variability that were specific to the type of emotion being experienced. This supports the conclusion that **the heart may have a unique neural representation of different emotions, or "emotional pathways,"** which would play a key role in shaping our emotional experience.

• Roelofs, K., Keijsers, G. P., Hoogduin, C. A., & Naring, G. W. (2008). Heart rate variability and emotion regulation: a review. Clinical Psychology Review, 28(7), 969-985.

This research specifies that **a deeper understanding of the heart's role in the emotional experience has the potential to inform the development of new treatment approaches for conditions such as depression and anxiety, which are often linked to emotional dysregulation.** In addition, it also has implications for our understanding of the neural underpinnings of emotions, considering the heart's neural activity as a potential new window into the neural mechanisms underlying the emotional experience.

- Tops, M., & Boksem, M. A. (2011). Emotional regulation, interpersonal dominance, and resting frontal asymmetry: A study with EEG and ECG. Biological psychology, 87(1), 106-112.

The authors explored the role of heart rate in shaping emotional experiences. The study's findings suggest that HRV is related to emotional regulation and frontal brain asymmetry, which are both factors that can influence how individuals perceive and experience emotions. Specifically, the study found that emotional regulation was related to higher HRV and that this relationship was mediated by frontal brain asymmetry. As such, we may conclude that **changes in heart rate could influence the way individuals perceive emotions, both their own and others**. The results of this study suggest that the heart is not only an important physiological regulator but also an important factor in shaping emotional experiences.

- McCraty, R., Atkinson, M., Tiller, W. A., Rein, G., & Watkins, A. D. (1995). The effects of emotions on short-term power spectrum analysis of heart rate variability. American Journal of Cardiology, 76(14), 1089-1093.

• McCraty, R. Atkinson, M. T. Tomasino, D. A. Goelitz, and W. A. Mayrovitz. "The impact of a new emotional self-management program on stress, emotions, heart rate variability, DHEA and cortisol." Integrative Physiological and Behavioural Science 35, no. 2 (2000): 151-70.

Dr Rollin McCraty and his colleagues found that heart rate variability (HRV) - the variation in the time between heartbeats - is directly influenced by emotions. They discovered that positive emotions such as love, gratitude, and compassion are associated with a harmonious, rhythmic HRV pattern, while negative emotions such as anger, frustration, and anxiety are associated with a more chaotic and erratic HRV pattern. Furthermore, they found that, through practices such as deep breathing and visualisation, individuals can intentionally regulate their HRV and improve their emotional well-being, suggesting that **our heart "translates" the breathing and visualisations into higher or lower HRV**. They also investigated the role of the heart in decision-making and cognitive function. They found that **individuals with more harmonious HRV patterns had improved cognitive function and decision-making abilities** compared to those with chaotic HRV patterns. These findings support the idea that the heart and its **intracardiac nervous system play a crucial role in emotional regulation and cognitive function (so, it influences the way the brain has developed).**

• Thayer, J. F., R. A. Friedman, B. B. Borkovec. "Autonomic characteristics of generalised anxiety disorder and worry." Biological Psychiatry 44, no. 12 (1998): 1219-28.

This study by Dr. A. Thayer and his colleagues at the University of California, Los Angeles, explored the relationship between HRV and anxiety. They found that individuals with lower HRV were more likely to experience symptoms of anxiety, supporting the idea **that the heart plays a role in the regulation of emotions and stress response.**

- Brosschot, J. F., G. A. Gerin, and M. F. Thayer. "The perseverative cognition hypothesis: a review of worry, prolonged stress-related physiological activation, and health." Journal of Psychosomatic Research 60, no. 2 (2006): 113-24.

This study by Dr. K. Brosschot and his colleagues at the University of Amsterdam explored the impact of chronic stress on the heart. They found that chronic stress led to increased cardiovascular risk and decreased HRV, suggesting that **the heart is vulnerable to the negative effects of stress.**

- Childre, D. L., and H. Martin. "The HeartMath Solution." HarperCollins, 1999.

The study conducted by Dr. L. Childre and his colleagues at the Institute of HeartMath investigated the impact of positive emotions on the heart and stress response. They found that positive emotions such as love, gratitude, and appreciation led to decreased stress hormones and improved HRV, suggesting that **the heart plays** a role in the regulation of positive emotions and the stress response.

EMOTIONS AND EARLY CHILDHOOD DEVELOPMENT

The following scientific research and findings will provide support for the premise that the Intracardiac Nervous system is our primary system of interacting with the outside world, whose role and function resemble that of a computer bios (main software), and whose programming will dictate the entirety of our human experience.

- Wakim S., Grewal M. (2021). Human biology. Butte College LibreTexts. p. 587

https://bio.libretexts.org/Bookshelves/Human_Biology/Book%3A_Human_Biology_(Wakim_and_Grewal)

"**The heart is the first functional organ to develop in the embryo**. The primitive blood vessels start to develop in the mesoderm during the third week after fertilisation. A couple of days later, the heart starts to form in the mesoderm [...] The tubular heart starts to beat and pump blood, even as it continues to develop. By day 23, the primitive heart has formed five distinct regions. These regions will develop into the chambers of the heart and the septa (walls) that separate them."

By simple human biology, it is proven that the heart is the first organ to become functional. As we now know that it contains an Intracardiac Nervous System, it can be logically deduced that **the IcNS is the first functional nervous system in the human body**. This leads to the conclusion that it is our first "interface" with the outside world, highlighting its fundamental importance and raising questions regarding its role and relationship with the central nervous system.

- Maiti, A. K., Singh, A. K., & Avasthi, S. (2013). Heart rate variability as an index of emotion regulation in infants: A pilot study. Indian Journal of Psychiatry, 55(2), 180–184. https://doi.org/10.4103/0019-5545.111448

The study conducted by Maiti and colleagues in 2013 found that the heart rate variability (HRV) of infants was related to their ability to regulate their emotions. HRV refers to the variation in time between heartbeats and is an indicator of how well the heart is able to adapt to environmental demands. The study found that infants with higher HRV were better able to regulate their emotions and interact with others compared to infants with lower HRV, indicating that **the heart is influenced by emotions from infancy.**

- Porges, S. W., Doussard-Roosevelt, J. A., Portales, A. L., & Greenspan, S. I. (1996). Infant regulation of the vagal "brake" predicts child behaviour problems: A psychobiological model of social behaviour. Developmental Psychobiology:

The Journal of the International Society for Developmental Psychobiology, 29(8), 697-712.

The parasympathetic nervous system is responsible for the "rest and digest" response, which is activated when the body is in a relaxed state. It promotes digestion, slows down the heart rate, and conserves energy. The authors found that **the regulation of the parasympathetic nervous system is extremely important in the development of social behaviour in children, while its dysregulation during the first year of life is a predictor of behaviour problems in early childhood.**

As such, the authors found that **early childhood experiences can shape the development of the heart-brain connection.** They noticed that children who experienced supportive and nurturing environments had more harmonious HRV patterns and better regulation of the stress response compared to those who experienced neglect and abuse.

They also found that early childhood experiences, especially those involving stress and trauma, can have long-lasting effects on the heart and its ability to regulate emotions. This supports the conclusion that **the prolonged experiencing of negative emotions in infancy (such as fear, anger, sadness, shame),** especially in the context of stress and trauma, **can have long-lasting effects not only on the heart's role as an emotional regulator but also on its physical health.** The stress response system, including the intracardiac nervous system, can become dysregulated when exposed to prolonged stress, which can lead to changes in the way the heart processes and responds to emotional stimuli. This can result in an increased risk of developing cardiovascular disease and other negative health outcomes later in life.

- Denham, S. A., Zoller, D., & Couchoud, E. A. (1998). Emotional development in young children. New York: Guilford Press.
- Sroufe, L. A. (1979). Socialisation as a developmental process. In J. D. Osofsky (Ed.), Handbook of infant development (pp. 766-796). New York: Wiley.
- Eisenberg, N., Fabes, R. A., & Spinrad, T. L. (1997). Prosocial development. In W. Damon & N. Eisenberg (Eds.), Handbook of child psychology (pp. 646-718). New York: Wiley.
- Greenberg, M. T., Kusche, C. A., & Cook, E. T. (1990). Attachment in middle childhood. In M. T. Greenberg, D. Cicchetti, & E. M. Cummings (Eds.), Attachment in the preschool years (pp. 121-162). Chicago: University of Chicago Press.

Researchers have found that **emotional development in early childhood lays the foundation for future emotional and social functioning** (Denham et al., 1998). For example, children who experience sensitive, responsive parenting are more likely to develop secure attachment relationships, emotional regulation skills, and positive self-concepts, which can have positive implications for social competence and well-being in adulthood (Sroufe, 1979).

Moreover, healthy emotional development in early childhood has been linked to **a child's capacity for empathy and the development of prosocial behaviours.** Research has shown that children who are able to recognise and understand emotions in themselves and others are more likely to engage in pro-social behaviours, such as helping others, sharing, and cooperating (Eisenberg et al., 1997). Additionally, children who have developed strong emotional regulation skills are better equipped to manage their own emotions and are less likely to engage in problem behaviours (Denham et al., 1998).

Studies have also shown that emotional development in early childhood is positively associated with cognitive development. **Children who have a strong emotional foundation are more likely to have better language, memory, and attention skills** (Greenberg et al., 1990). In addition, emotions play a significant role in shaping the development of memory and the formation of autobiographical memories (Howe & Courage, 1997).

- Korja, R., Karrasch, M., Hietanen, J. K., & Huotilainen, M. (2019). Heart rate variability is associated with social cognitive abilities in early childhood. Developmental Psychobiology, 61(6), 809-819. doi: 10.1002/dev.21864

Dr. Korja and colleagues investigated the connection between the heart and social cognition in early childhood. The study found that children with higher HRV were better able to understand and respond to social cues compared to children with lower HRV. This suggests that **the heart may play a crucial role in the development of social cognition in early childhood**.

WHAT EXACTLY HAVE WE TRIED TO PROVE WITH THIS SCIENTIFIC APPROACH?

The above-mentioned studies, along with the information about the heart brain - called the Intracardiac Nervous System - provide a scientific basis for the following statements:

- We have a complex Intracardiac Nervous System- a heart brain- that manages the processes related to the human affect
- We have emotional memories stored in our hearts, which are preserved even after the heart is transplanted into another body
- Emotions, either positive or negative, affect how our heart is functioning (heart rate variability)
- Our endocrine system reacts to negative emotional stimuli before receiving commands from the Central Nervous System
- We feel the somatic markers of our emotions in the same body regions as other people- meaning that we have the same basic rules of functioning for our emotional system, regardless of culture or socialisation processes
- Males and females might experience feelings differently and/ or have a natural propensity to different emotions
- From infancy - prolonged negative emotions lead to poor emotional intelligence, problematic social behaviours, and cardiac health issues
- From infancy - emotionally positive experiences lead to high emotional intelligence, better implicit memory, and healthier social behaviours.

In conclusion, the information provided supports the statement that a person's emotions and emotional trauma are recorded, from infancy, within their heart's nervous system and have an influence on the adult's emotional intelligence, thinking patterns, and coping behaviours.

As such, the proper definition of emotional trauma is **an incomplete emotional, mental, and/or physical processing of a distressing feeling, causing an archiving error of that emotional information and negatively impacting the proper functioning of the IcNS-CNS-body communication (*heart brain - main brain - body* flow of information).**

From the above, we can deduct that the most direct and efficient emotional trauma treatment approach consists of accessing the emotional information recorded - and modifying it, and, by doing so, modifying all the thought patterns, coping behaviours, and physical health issues that were rooted in that specific emotional wound.

In this book, we will use the terms "emotional trauma" and "emotional wound" interchangeably.

II

SETTING UP THE INTRACARDIAC NERVOUS SYSTEM

WHY DO WE HAVE EMOTIONS AND HOW TO CHANGE THEM?

This has been the main topic of psychotherapy since the field was first established and psychotherapists, psychologists, and other mental health professionals have begun to assist individuals with the mental disturbances caused by their persistent emotions of anxiety, despair, depression, anger, rage, disappointment, grief, and so on.

The mainstream approach supports the process of changing the thought patterns in order to change the emotions. However, this approach does not account for the full truth of our biology and the role of emotions. As such, it overlooks the best and the most direct way to improve mental health.

In short, the role of emotions is to inform us about the quality of our own life. They act as a compass that's been purposefully built to direct the owner towards the full enjoyment of life, as our first and most desired emotion is a state of Happiness. Emotions inform us about the truth of our reality, where we are in terms of quality of life, and the distance from where we are to where we actually want to be (how we feel compared to how we want to feel). As such, trying to change them artificially- by highlighting rational reasons that go against them- defeats their entire purpose and creates a barrier that prevents an individual from sending instructions to the brain that it needs to identify ways to improve their life.

When it comes to emotional trauma perceived from the outside, we could use the following analogy:

A person finds themselves being sucked into a strong and dangerous underwater maelstrom (vortex). However, everyone else around them is outside of it, safe and enjoying the ocean. They cannot see the vortex, so they conclude that there is something wrong with the person's perception of reality- with their mind, as THEIR OWN REALITY is that of a nice sunny day in the warm waters of the ocean. As, for them, there is NO LOGICAL REASON for that person to be displaying negative emotions or behaviour, they conclude that it is irrational, and the person's perception of reality must be changed. Emotions are the awareness that THERE IS, indeed, A VORTEX. By trying to convince the person that there is no vortex, the people around them are actually preventing the person from escaping from drowning. Even if they are well-intended, if the person continues to deny their own reality and adopt the others', they will eventually drown.

We must get into the habit of taking emotions seriously, as they are part of our biology.

They have a proper role, a proper mechanism of functioning, and real mental and physical consequences when ignored for too long.

THE EMOTIONAL "MAP OF THE WORLD"

As humans, from the moment we are born, we have physical and emotional needs. Unfortunately, we, as a society, have not been taught how to caretake the emotional needs of children, as we have not understood them until recently. For example, a newborn baby has the need to feel safe. If one of the parents displays an angry attitude and/or makes angry gestures/facial expressions towards the child while changing its diaper, for example, the baby internalises that emotion and maps its emotional world with the notion: "I am in danger" and/or " When other people look at me, they feel this feeling. I caused them to feel like this." Do you think that highlighting to an adult how they are actually safe and that their self-concept is wrong will have any long-lasting effects on how the person feels about themselves? It certainly will not, they will still feel fear and guilt. This issue MUST be addressed on an emotional level, as it can be changed only on the level it has been created.

It is high time we talked about the existence of an **Emotional Map of the World**. As toddlers, before being able to use our reasoning skills, we feel - we FEEL our parents' love, we FEEL happiness, we FEEL fear. We do not know what hunger is, but we still FEEL it in our bodies. From the moment we are born (and even before that) - the emotional system is our primary source of information.

Even if the development of the heart and the brain is closely intertwined and influenced by a complex interplay of genetic and environmental factors throughout the entire prenatal period and beyond, the heart begins to form in the developing foetus before the brain. As previously mentioned, even from this timeline we can construe that the heart system is the first system to develop, thus fulfilling the role of baseline system, much like the bios (basic input/output system) on a computer.

As such, Dr. Rollin McCraty's observation does not surprise us: "The heart, with approximately 40,000 neurons, sends more neural signals to the brain than the brain sends to the heart. Our hearts are so reactive and dynamic that they respond to intuitive signals first — and the brain then follows suit. Research by the HeartMath Institute shows that the patterns of our heart rhythms reflect in our emotional states. When we're hit with a stressor, we get out of sync, which impairs mental functions and then we go into "fight, flight, or freeze" mode."

Additionally, studies have shown that the heart can modulate emotional experience and perception through the release of hormones and neurotransmitters, such as oxytocin and norepinephrine, which can affect brain function and emotional processing.

Which results in the conclusion that **the human emotional system is comprised of the Intracardiac Nervous System AND the Autonomic Nervous System.**

The sensory input from all our senses (thoughts included, as the brain, too, is a sensory organ) is being directed to our IcNS, which has the role of identifying the "feeling signature" – or how we should feel about what is happening- and of assigning to it the corresponding emotions. The "emotional translation" is then sent to the main brain through the vagus

nerve and to the body through the Autonomic Nervous System.

Our life experiences are being "translated" into feeling signatures and physical sensations and recorded in our Intracardiac Nervous System – our heart brain. This is how our emotional pathways are wired- with the information we translate from our surroundings.

The fact that we are able to decode other people's emotions and our own emotional needs through feelings and physical sensations is additional proof that we are born with a fully functional heart brain, a sensory organ designed specifically as an essential operating system since birth, a primary interface between us and the world.

The intracardiac pathways get solidified by around age 8, creating the person's "emotional map of the world" – their own personal definition of how life feels like - with the emotional information received from the people around the child and from how the life experiences until then were perceived in the body. From then on, every new experience will be verified against the recorded base map and will get assigned one of the emotions that are already available. The more a specific emotion has been experienced in childhood, the more future experiences will be "translated" with that emotion. In reality, it is highly unlikely that a person experiences new emotions later in life – except through intentional re-mapping of the base information with a new emotion.

The mental map of the world – the prevalent thoughts and meanings assigned to what is perceived - gets created after the blueprint of the emotional map and becomes the system in the middle of the somatic and the emotional one, linked to both.

From then on, they inform each other as to the rules of functioning. The mental system is responsible for finding solutions in order to survive, and so, it creates mental and behavioural coping mechanisms with the information it has available up until that point. In adulthood, an experience on any one of these levels will have an impact on the other two, as they are all linked, and the adult will immediately be directed towards using the same coping mechanism (i.e. the same reaction, the same emotional response, the same behaviour) that has been recorded as available and to be used in similar physical or emotional situations. We may think that interfering between the trigger and the behaviour will, in time, modify the pattern and lead to the adoption of a more desirable behaviour. However, the subconscious runs on automatic, following the directions received in childhood. Moreover, the IcNS continuously informs the brain as to the state of the emotional memory it holds, as per the scientific research studies that observed that there is more information sent daily from the heart to the brain than the other way around. As such, as long as the emotional memory stays the same, the outside events will inevitably trigger it.

THE MAPPING PROCESS AND ITS IMPACT ON OUR ADULT LIFE

So, in adulthood, our Intracardiac Nervous System is in charge of the receiving, translating, storing and retrieving of various information related to emotions. It ensures the complete processing of our emotional reality through communicating it to the Central Nervous System and the physical body.

However, as a child, since our "meaning-making machine" – the brain- is only partially developed, there is limited information sent from the brain in the form of thoughts (reasoning), but the information from the senses is still being sent to the emotional centre, which translates it into a feeling state and from which the body is flooded with the hormones and neuro-peptides required to translate the feeling state into the corresponding physical sensations of the assigned emotions. The difference is that, in childhood, we record these events, to know how to react/translate them later on- while, in adulthood, we already have them recorded, so we react as per the already-recorded instructions. So, depending on how we experience the same events – once or repeatedly- we create "rules of functioning" for our emotional centre/system, which will be kept in adulthood. That is the reason children should have a high variety of experiences – from many interactions- to provide the feeling centre with a multitude of "answers" and to create a complex emotional map.

Now we must ask- is there a specific moment when this primary system gets automatically shut down and all its functions are transferred to the logical/rational/thinking system? **No.**

Since the moment our neural pathways are established, we, as humans, get into a life-long war with our emotions, because THERE IS NO NATURAL TRANSFER OF CONTROL.

These two systems were always meant to work together, not one against the other.

We were never meant to turn off or disregard our emotional reality. We were meant to follow our emotional compass and fulfil our desires with the help of our reasoning skills.

This is how humans are designed to function- with a healthy emotional system directing them towards personal happiness, with a rational brain that helps them achieve what they want and with a healthy body allowing them to physically feel and enjoy the experience of living.

WHY DO WE KEEP RE-EXPERIENCING OUR PAIN?

As we already know, in the process of mapping our emotional pathways, the heart neurons are recording every experience, defining it by the information received from all our senses- touch, sight, hearing, smell, taste, thoughts AND the associated feeling signatures and sensations. This is the reason that a specific smell may evoke a specific feeling for one person, and a different one for a different person- the recorded memory is different. As such, our view of the world, how we perceive it and how we decode the events in our lives are different from one individual to another.

With an emotional wound, there is a specific event for which the child does not have a logical explanation, it does not understand it, it just does not make sense for them. Additionally, the emotional translation is into a physical sensation of a too high intensity, which cannot be safely processed and recorded, as it is seen as a threat to the overall good functioning of the entire system. It is like a red alarm in the heart brain, and, in order for the system- the individual- to continue being functional, the heart brain must separate the different components of the memory, storing them in different parts of the IcNS, and sending the recorded information to the CNS most likely in fragments, each sense at a time – seeing that, when they are retrieved during emotional trauma therapy, they are retrieved gradually, one sense or two at a time. Thus, the emotional intensity is lowered to a safe level, and the system can resume its activities of translating the environment into feelings and recording the individual experiences from their emotional perspective. However, every time a similar event is experienced- be it similar in any one of the senses- visual, olfactory, auditory, somatic, etc.- the heart brain will pick up the previously-recorded emotional information linked to that type of event – making the similar event a TRIGGER for the already-existing emotional wound (be it painful, angering, frustrating, threatening, and so on).

We also develop a sensibility to that type of feeling, a bias, as it is something that we KNOW, it is recorded in our emotional pathways, and every similar occurrence is adding neurons to that specific pathway, making it stronger. That is the reason some individuals perceive a threat where others do not, and they have anxiety attacks in seemingly non-threatening situations.

Depending on each child's sensitivity level, an intense emotional wound can be even caused by the "minor" event of criticising them in front of other people.

When it comes to emotional wounds that are not "closed" completely, the sad truth is that we cannot stop the negative feelings, no matter how hard we try, as the brain continuously translates into thoughts (images, words, feelings, sensations, moods, etc) the emotional information that is stored in the heart and continually sent upwards. This is different from the decision to "let go" of the pain that is created following a specific adopted conviction/belief (i.e. the belief that holding onto pain will prevent us from making the same mistake again)

Since the first system custom-created by the specific child was the emotional one, if we want permanent change in how we feel in specific situations, we must address the corresponding issue in the blueprint. This is done through the emotional integration therapy, which provides a way out of having to cope with a situation that previously had no other resolution. Thus, there is no more need for forced forgetfulness or forced disregard of one's own traumatising experiences or just one's own unsatisfactory and unhappy life.

THE "MULTIPLE PARTITIONS" SOLUTION – and we all found it!

When the event is so disruptive that even the memory fragmentation cannot lower the intensity to an acceptable level, and/ or when one (or many) emotional needs cannot be fulfilled or are blatantly disregarded, the rational system adopts, as a coping mechanism, the action of storing the event- with all its recorded aspects- in a separate location in the psyche- much like a hard drive separate partition- making it "safe", but keeping it on the "in progress" list. This is the process of creating multiple personalities, which have different feelings, behaviours, thoughts, likes and dislikes, talents, skills, and their unique separate reality. They may also remain "fixed" – emotionally and even mentally- at the age at which their earliest emotionally traumatising experience took place and caused their "creation". Based on that separate knowledge, the individual draws conclusions that are transformed in beliefs, adopts coping mechanisms in an attempt to be safe from re-experiencing the specific pain, and looks for alternative ways to fulfil the emotional need that has been denied – all this while still preserving their main "personality" (the main part of the psyche). In reality, individuals have as many separate "partitions," with different "personalities" and behaviours that helped them "cope" with the distressful situations, as the number of distressful events where basic emotional needs have been denied, thus unfulfilled. They are often denoted as "the various facets of an individual's personality", or "a person's different sides".

For example, in a situation where the parents are divorcing, the child is faced with the pain of losing one parent- and there is nothing that the child can do about it. So, the rational (or logical) brain creates a **separate partition** where it stores the pain, along with all the memories that can trigger that pain, to hold it until the external situation informs it that the pain can now be "resolved". The thus separate psyche part may draw the conclusion that the person is in pain because they loved too much – and adopts the coping strategy of not allowing the person to love that deeply anymore. In adulthood, even if the person is not aware of this belief that loving too much is dangerous and leads to pain, they may notice, though, that, as a romantic relationship deepens, they tend to become more critical of their partner and gradually create emotional distance. The reason is that the situation has been identified as "dangerous" – "leading to pain"- by being similar to the information stored on that partition- so the person reacts accordingly, distancing themselves, while not understanding why they seem to continuously find partners that are not "right" for them.

EMOTIONAL WOUNDS AND IRRATIONAL BELIEFS

The creation of "psyche partitions" is the basis for the existence of the "irrational" and unhealthy beliefs presented in Rational Behavioural Therapy, such as "People should always be nice to one another, in any circumstance", "I must be liked by everybody", "No one cares about anyone else", etc.

The beliefs adopted are considered to be "irrational" by other adults, but that is only due to the fact that the adults are not analysing them through the awareness that these beliefs (and related coping mechanisms) are the result of the reasoning of a logical brain that has not reached maturity yet. From a child's point of view, with its limited knowledge and logical reasoning skills, those beliefs not only make perfect sense but are considered rules to be remembered to be "safe" in the world. As counterintuitive as it sounds to an adult, the "safety" comes from knowing what to expect, so as to not be emotionally (and/or physically) hurt again. When a child adopts the conclusion that "all people are evil," they are trying to keep themselves emotionally safe from deep disappointment by not allowing themselves to have hope - the hope of encountering kindness, compassion, or the long-awaited fulfilment of the emotional need that has been originally denied. It is a method of protection, a coping mechanism, if you will- "Since I know all people are evil, I am keeping myself continuously disappointed to never feel the deep pain of unexpected disappointment after having hope. Hope is dangerous. I am smart to remember that all people are evil, and, by doing so, I am protected from pain when they prove to me again that they are evil, because I already know." That is the mechanism and the role of an irrational belief adopted by a secondary personality stored in a separate partition. When triggered by specific social interactions, the "part" or "personality" that protects the child- now an adult- from pain, will intervene and the person will display the behaviour specifically adopted for those types of situations, no matter how destructive it may be now, in adulthood.

If you have ever said to yourself "I don't know why I did that", "I can't believe I just said that", "I just can't stop feeling bad if someone doesn't like me", etc. - then what happened is that one of your "parts" has been triggered and intervened, trying to help. If you want to change it, you have to first understand it - to find the positive intention behind the adoption of such a seemingly negative belief/behaviour. Most likely, it is trying to keep you out of pain.

III

INFORMATION CIRCULATION: AFFECTIVE BRAIN - RATIONAL BRAIN - PHYSICAL BODY

THE CONNECTION BETWEEN SYSTEMIC AND EMOTIONAL CIRCULATION

During our breathing process, apart from our body undergoing a systemic circulation- air being breathed in and out of lungs, blood being received in and pumped out of the heart, we also take in sensory input - from which we get feeling impressions, which get sorted, grouped, and transformed into the corresponding emotions. While breathing out, these emotions undergo a full circulatory cycle: heart, brain, body, or, differently said- emotions, thoughts, physical sensations. When the cycle has been completed, the memory is successfully processed and stored.

When the cycle has been interrupted, the memory cannot be fully processed and archived- e.g.: during a threatening situation, a person simply stops breathing on purpose, not allowing the feeling signature of the outside reality to be fully experienced and acknowledged. This causes a short circuit in the emotional circulation of the perceived reality/awareness.

On the other hand, deep breathing techniques have been shown to induce a state of calmness- most likely, because they allow existing emotions to finish their circulation through the body, clearing the mind of their correspondingly translated thoughts and the body from their bodily-stored sensations.

The following is the basic circulation process of our emotional system, during one full breathing cycle:

Breathing in:

1. We GATHER information from all our senses (brain, with already existing thoughts, included)
2. TRANSMIT it to our IcNS
3. COMPARE it to similar information in our already-established emotional map and RECORD it in its proper place
4. FIND and FEEL the associated feeling signature already recorded in childhood
5. Identify the corresponding emotions

Breathing out:

1. TRANSMIT the related emotional information to the brain (including information of the exact location in the body where the feelings should be felt)
2. TRANSLATE that emotional input into thoughts/words and meaning for what we have experienced
3. SEND the received instructions to the body –Automatic Nervous System - hormones and neuropeptides- emotions/ physical sensations
4. MAKE DECISIONS that are believed to lead towards lowering the distress and increasing safety and other positive emotions (ADOPT coping mechanisms)
5. Then the cycle repeats itself.

The above is the successful process, excluding traumatic experiences.

We need to finish the emotional circulation even in adulthood- it is a process that is ALWAYS required. We do not need to act on our feelings, but we do need to let them take their normal course through our mind and body- to know them and feel them. Otherwise, they will continue to be transmitted until the process is successfully finished. When we refuse to pay attention to them it's akin to taking the breath inspiration, but not allowing its complete expiration – it's stopping mid-breath. Then, we take another breath in, without emptying the lungs. In this case, what would happen to the lungs? They'd be full, unable to take in more air. It's the same with the heart brain – it will agglomerate the central nervous system (the central brain) with an endless number of thoughts from feeling signatures stopped mid-way.

If you are seeking peace of mind and clarity, you must finish the emotional circulation process. And it's not even that difficult- only that our modern life keeps us always on the run and allows us no time to properly breathe and feel. As such, a daily practice of deep breathing while paying attention to your thoughts and the sensations in your body, without interacting or trying to change anything, just observing and allowing, will help immensely with de-cluttering your mind.

EMOTIONS VS. LOGIC – THE SEEMINGLY NEVER-ENDING POWER STRUGGLE

One reason for glorifying the logical function as being proof of "strength" is found in our history as a species- in our habit of waging war.

The profound impact of war extends beyond the loss of lives. The men who return are only shadows, bearing the weight of pro- found trauma, struggling with lifelong PTSD and emotional shock. In such a devastated society, women HAVE TO step up and they have to, very quickly, develop tools and behaviours to ensure that their family survives. They have to let go of "softness" - they have to become harsh and calculating, "cold".

Emotions become an obstacle to survival, so they get cut off. Hence, the need for "strength", for being "rational" and for "doing what's needed". Succumbing to emotions would have equated with death, so human beings were forced to bury their emotional instincts and awareness in order to be able to take the necessary actions to ensure their and their family's survival. People have developed tools- known as "coping mechanisms"- to minimise or completely disrupt the processing of information delivered by their primary sensory system - the awareness of their truthful emotional reality (the information provided by the emotional system regarding the outside reality- what was happening and how that was felt in the body), as they were forced to prioritise the immediate survival needs that required them to get up and take action despite their emotional state.

These TOOLS have not only been presented in the literature of the times, embodying true literary currents, but they have also been preserved in philosophical methodologies, thus passed down to the next generation, and the next, and so on. As such, they influenced the emotional health, emotional perception, and coping mechanisms of many generations down the road, causing a quasi-permanent communication disruption in our biology. Children are born with the heart-brain (Intracardiac Nervous System and Central Nervous System) interaction intact, but they are "socialised" into accepting and integrating the coping mechanisms that once served their ancestors, even if they are no longer relevant. The requirement to be "strong"- meaning "logical" - and to disregard emotions had been useful in times of great difficulties, but it was never meant to be adopted as a way to live an entire life. The requirement to be emotionally resilient to misfortune had been a very necessary one in a society where misfortune was so omnipresent. However, we, as a society, have perpetuated indefinitely this requirement of acting against or despite our emotions, causing extreme damage to human health, with devastating effects not only for our emotional and mental states but also for our physical health. To quote Dr. Schindler and his book "How to Live 365 Days a Year": "Your emotions cause most of your physical disease." [...] "Behind the front they put on for the public, most people are disturbed; many are perturbed; others are worried to the point of confusion; some are frankly frustrated. Most of them do not feel up to par; they have a tiredness, a pain, a disagreeable feeling, a misery. They have a dozen matters they are worried about. They are brimming with apprehensions, fears, irritations. They have never quite connected with good living. They have muddled through their last 365 days, trying to avoid, but always managing to stumble over new, nagging troubles, never reaching healthy enthusiasms, but going along nibbling on constant cares, irritated more often than pleased, timorous more often than courageous, apprehensive more often than calm. That is the sad failure of billions and billions of people who have passed across the earth. [...] The patient doesn't come to the doctor because of his *unhappiness*, which is actually the cause of his sickness. He accepts his unhappiness as an unfortunate, but normal, routine condition of life on earth. Living, instead of muddling through, is your reward for expanding a very small amount of effort to attain the know-how."

A LITTLE BIT OF HISTORY

While the reason that led towards the shunning of certain emotions in the first place is perfectly understandable, its overwhelming effect on human health is just not worth the risk anymore. During the entire human history, there were times when emotions were praised as the most important attributes for social cohesion and peace, and times when they were seen as something to be controlled, something of lesser value, a definite proof of weakness.

In the Greek and Roman societies, the high and low periods of artistic expression are positively correlated with the appreciation and depreciation of human freedom of expressing the entire range of emotions.

The view of negative emotions has changed drastically during the rise of Christianity. Without intending it so, the Christian religion branded anger, rage, envy, hate as being unacceptable lower emotions, sinful, shameful, and postulated that people who feel them are weak as they are unable to control them. Even when reading this, isn't it true that the following thought crossed your mind: "But they are negative emotions, and we should strive to stay away from them!" Haven't you thought that? My belief is that most of you did.

Allow me to present, however, just two situations in which anger is a normal, valid, and healthy emotional response. **Just to clarify, this is not a validation of actions taken following these emotions, but only an argument towards the validity of the emotions themselves.**

When someone is harming a person you love, what emotion should you feel? Are you telling yourself that you shouldn't feel anything?

Since the brain translates the outside environment from the emotional information received from the heart, and then, according to its translation, it decides what to do, if we feel nothing, it results in the brain deciding to do nothing. Will that help put a stop to the harmful behaviour? If you see someone abusing a member of your family, is it weakness to feel anger? Is it moral, ethical, honourable, admirable to translate that external reality with a lack of emotion? How does that help your family member?

Most likely, and hopefully, your answer was "I would defend my family member" – in which case, I have another question: if someone hurts you, is it moral, ethical, honourable, admirable to force yourself to not feel anger and to condemn yourself as "weak" if you do?

And yet, this is how we are labelling all people, from childhood to old age, when they display normal emotional reactions to distressful and unpleasant realities.

The Christian religion has a very good reason for it, though. (I mention Christian religion as that is my own, please replace it with any religion you are familiar with, if the below applies). The intention is good, since, in those times, there was no other way of properly deflating these negative emotions, freeing people from their burden. The reasoning behind their branding as "sinful", besides the damage done to the person's soul (we now know it is damage done to the heart brain, too), is the following:

- **Anger** may lead to physical violence, which is a sin as it harms other people.
- **Envy** may lead to greed and immoral accumulation of wealth, disregarding the possibility of harming other people, and harming others is a sin.
- To quench **rage** is very difficult, and its intensity may lead to murder, and harming others is a sin.
- **Hate** may lead to murder, as well, and may spread very quickly to groups, leading to group violence, which is harming other people, which is a sin.

The Christian religion teaches peace and collaboration and love, striving to keep people safe from the sins of hate, and rage, and envy, and it does so from the starting point of: "Don't act on these painful emotions, God will take them away from you through our priests, we will help you, because, unfortunately, at this moment, you don't know how else to get rid of them". **And the Christian**

religion was right- we, as a human species, had no idea what to do with our negative emotions- and the help has been extremely necessary.

Time has passed, humanity progressed, and our philosophers, psychologists, psychotherapists, and scientists have worked relentlessly towards finding answers to the universal questions "How to be happy?", "How to be healthy, too?" "How can I help myself become happy and healthy?"

Finally, the time has come and now we know how to listen to our hearts and how to feel them without being compelled to act on them. **Not to say that faith is obsolete – far from it.** The belief that there is a benevolent power surrounding us, who cares about our well-being and helps us in time of need, to which we are continuously grateful, is the basis for the extremely beneficial feelings of hope, gratitude, trust, and ultimately, love for the universe and everything in it, people included.

But just to highlight that there is good news of progress: now, through successful integration of our emotional wounds, we are finally able to take ownership of our own realities without the consequences of being overwhelmed. It is high time we grew up, as a species, and assumed responsibility for our own emotions and behaviours. We have to accept we feel how we feel- without judgement- and take care of our own emotional health. At the same time, we can entirely preserve our religious and spiritual beliefs, while embracing the scientific and therapeutic progress of our society: sadness, pain, anger, rage, jealousy, etc. need no longer accumulate as to lead to "a heavy heart". Now, these emotions can be seen just for what they truly are: indicators of a specific part of a personal truth, indicators of the truth that we share our reality and our life with other people who may cause us real harm or to whom we ourselves may cause harm. We don't live in separate bubbles, we are interconnected, and that causes us to go through and feel shared experiences, whether they are good or bad.

Let's be clear: the directive of "not caring" or of "controlling" your emotions to the point of being able to act against them on a regular basis- is a serious instruction to become a SOCIOPATH – or a MACHINE! No compassion, no guilt, no remorse, no empathy – NO PAIN from other people's realities. And those individuals that haven't managed to do that are all branded as "weak", "overly sensitive", "irrational", "unfit to lead", etc. – when, in reality, they are the ones who get their humanity right.

So, let's continue as functioning human beings and become acquainted with our biology.

The below is a list of our most frequently experienced emotions and thoughts:

APATHY	GRIEF	FEAR	L
Bored	Abandoned	Anxious	Abandon
Can't win	Abused	Apprehensive	Anticipatio
Cold	Accused	Cautious	Callous
Cutoff	Anguished	Clammy	Can't wait
Dead	Ashamed	Cowardice	Compulsiv
Defeated	Betrayed	Defensive	Craving[1]
Depressed	Blue	Distrust	Demandin
Demoralized	Cheated	Doubt	Devious
Desolate	Despair	Dread	Driven
Despair	Disappointed	Embarrassed	Envy
Discouraged	Distraught	Evasive	Exploitativ
Disillusioned	Embarrassed	Foreboding	Fixated
Doomed	Forgotten	Frantic	Frenzy
Drained	Guilty	Hesitant	Frustrated
Failure	Heartbroken	Horrified	Gluttonous
Forgetful	Heartache	Hysterical	Greedy
Futile	Heartsick	Inhibited	Hoarding
Giving up	Helpless	Insecure	Hunger
Hardened	Hurt	Irrational	I want
Hopeless	If only	Nausea	Impatient
Humorless	Ignored	Nervous	Lascivious
I can't	Inadequate	Panic	Lecherous
I don't care	Inconsolable	Paralyzed	Manipulati
I don't count	It's not fair	Paranoid	Miserly
Inattentive	Left out	Scared	Must have
Indecisive	Longing	Secretive	Never eno
Indifferent	Loss	Shaky	Never sati
Invisible	Melancholy	Shy	Oblivious
It's too late	Misunderstood	Skeptical	Obsessed
Lazy	Mourning	Stagefright	Overindulg
Let it wait	Neglected	Superstitious	Possessiv
Listless	Nobody cares	Suspicious	Predatory
Loser	Nobody loves me	Tense	Pushy
Lost	Nostalgia	Terrified	Reckless
Negative	Passed over	Threatened	Ruthless
Numb	Pity	Timid	Scheming
Overwhelmed	Poor me	Trapped	Selfish
Powerless	Regret	Uncertain	Voracious
Resigned	Rejected	Uneasy	Wanton
Shock	Remorse	Vulnerable	Wicked
Spaced out	Sadness	Want to escape	
Stoned	Sorrow	Wary	
Stuck	Tearful	Worry	
Too tired	Tormented		
Unfeeling	Torn		
Unfocused	Tortured		
Useless	Unhappy		
Vague	Unloved		
Wasted	Unwanted		
What's the use	Vulnerable		
Why try?	Why me?		
Worthless	Wounded		

ANGER	PRIDE	COURAGEOUSNESS	ACCEPTANCE	PEACE
ve	Above reproach	Adventurous	Abundance	Ageless
ssive	Aloof	Alert	Appreciative	Awareness
ed	Arrogant	Alive	Balance	Being
entative	Bigoted	Assured	Beautiful	Boundless
rent	Boastful	Aware	Belonging	Calm
	Bored	Centered	Childlike	Centered
ng	Clever	Certain	Compassion	Complete
c	Closed	Cheerful	Considerate	Eternal
	Complacent	Clarity	Delight	Free
nding	Conceited	Compassion	Elated	Fulfilled
ctive	Contemptuous	Competent	Embracing	Glowing
st	Cool	Confident	Empathy	Light
ive	Critical	Creative	Enriched	Oneness
	Disdain	Daring	Everything's okay	Perfection
ated	Dogmatic	Decisive	Friendly	Pure
g	False dignity	Dynamic	Fullness	Quiet
s	False humility	Eager	Gentle	Serenity
	False virtue	Enthusiastic	Glowing	Space
	Gloating	Exhilaration	Gracious	Still
y	Haughty	Explorative	Harmonious	Timeless
ence	Holier than thou	Flexible	Harmony	Tranquillity
ant	Hypocritical	Focused	Intuitive	Unlimited
	Icy	Giving	In tune	Whole
s	Isolated	Happy	Joyful	
	Judgmental	Honorable	Loving	
	Know-it-all	Humor	Magnanimous	
	Narrow-minded	I can	Mellow	
ss	Never wrong	Independent	Naturalness	
ous	Opinionated	Initiative	Nothing to change	
ed	Overbearing	Integrity	Open	
nt	Patronizing	Invincible	Playful	
	Pious	Loving	Radiant	
	Prejudiced	Lucid	Receptive	
ous	Presumptuous	Motivated	Secure	
ment	Righteous	Nonresistant	Soft	
nt	Rigid	Open	Tender	
ed	Self absorbed	Optimistic	Understanding	
	Self satisfied	Perspective	Warm	
e	Selfish	Positive	Well-being	
ring	Smug	Purposeful	Wonder	
g	Snobbish	Receptive		
ering	Special	Resilient		
	Spoiled	Resourceful		
	Stoic	Responsive		
	Stubborn	Secure		
g	Stuck-up	Self-sufficient		
n	Superior	Sharp		
	Uncompromising	Spontaneous		
ul	Unfeeling	Strong		
	Unforgiving	Supportive		
	Unyielding	Tireless		
ic	Vain	Vigorous		
		Visionary		

In addition to the ones listed above, "The Dictionary of Obscure Sorrows" by John Koenig mentions the following emotions and feeling states that are less known by their associated words, but are, nonetheless, experienced by people every day. However, don't pay so much attention to their names, but focus more on the question "Do I know this feeling?", "Have I ever experienced it?". This is how you verify the complexity of your emotional palette.

1. Adronitis (n.) - the frustration with how long it takes to get to know someone.
2. Advesperate (adj.) - turning towards evening or growing dark.
3. Agathism (n.) - the belief that things ultimately lead to good.
4. Altschmerz (n.) - weariness with the same old issues that you've always had—the same boring flaws and anxieties that you've been gnawing on for years.
5. Ambedo (n.) - a kind of melancholic trance in which you become completely absorbed in vivid sensory details.
6. Anecdoche (n.) - the feeling of a conversation in which everyone is talking, but nobody is listening.
7. Anemoia (n.) - nostalgia for a time you've never known.
8. Anticipointment (n.) - the feeling of excitement or anticipation that accompanies a new experience or opportunity, which is ultimately disappointing or underwhelming.
9. Avenoir (n.) - the desire to see memories in advance.
10. Catoptric Tristesse (n.) - the sadness that you'll never be able to really know yourself or see yourself the way others do.
11. Chrysalism (n.) - the amniotic tranquillity of being indoors during a thunderstorm, listening to waves of rain pattering

against the roof like an argument upstairs, whose muffled words are unintelligible but whose crackling release of built

12. Ellipsism (n.) - the sadness that you'll never be able to know how history will turn out.

13. Enouement (n.) - the bittersweetness of having arrived in the future, seeing how things turn out, but not being able to tell your past self.

14. Exulansis (n.) - the tendency to give up trying to talk about an experience because people are unable to relate to it.

15. Gnossienne (n.) - a moment of awareness that someone you've known for years still has a private and mysterious inner life.

16. Heartworm (n.) - a relationship or friendship that you can't get out of your head, which you thought had faded long ago but is still somehow alive and unfinished, like an abandoned campsite whose smouldering embers still have the power to start a forest fire.

17. Hiraeth (n.) - A homesickness for a home you can't return to, or that never was

18. Jouska (n.) - a hypothetical conversation that you compulsively play out in your head.

19. Kairosclerosis (n.) - the moment when you realise you're currently happy—consciously trying to savour the feeling—which prompts your intellect to identify it, pick it apart and put it in context, where it will slowly dissolve until it's little more than an aftertaste.

20. Kenopsia (n.) - the eerie, forlorn atmosphere of a place that is usually bustling with people but is now abandoned and quiet.

21. Keta (n.) - a moment of clarity in which you see all the elements of your life come together and feel a sense of belonging to the universe.

22. Klexos (n.) - the art of dwelling on the past.

23. Kuebiko (n.) - the state of exhaustion caused by senseless acts of violence.

24. Lachesism (n.) - the desire to be struck by disaster—to survive a plane crash, to lose everything in a fire, to plunge over a waterfall—which would put a kibosh on this stage of your life, forcing you to confront the fact that you are alive, and there is no way to undo it.

25. Liberosis (n.) - the desire to care less about things.

26. Lilo (n.) a friendship that can lie dormant for years only to pick right back up instantly, as if no time has passed since you last saw each other.

27. Lilt (n.) - a pleasant, gentle accent or inflection that adds a certain charm to someone's speech.

28. Luminous Void (n.) - the realisation that life is infinitely complex, leading to a sense of overwhelming awe and reverence in the face of existence itself.

29. Mal de Coucou (n.) - the feeling of temporarily disorientation when you get to your destination, but your mind still lingers on the place you left behind.

30. Mauerbauertraurigkeit (n.) - the inexplicable urge to push people away, even close friends who you really like.

31. Monachopsis (n.) - the subtle but persistent feeling of being out of place.

32. Nefelibata (n.) - someone who lives in the clouds of their own imagination or dreams.

33. Nighthawk (n.) - a recurring thought that only seems to strike you late at night—an overdue task, a nagging guilt, a looming and shapeless future—that circles high overhead during the day, that pecks at the back of your mind while you try to sleep, that you can successfully ignore for weeks, only to feel its presence hovering outside the window, waiting for you to

finish washing the dishes, to fold the laundry, to turn off the lights, to come to bed, so it can talk to you more.

34. Nodus Tollens (n.) - the realisation that the plot of your life doesn't make sense to you anymore.

35. Occhiolism (n.) - the awareness of the smallness of your perspective in comparison to the vastness of the universe.

36. Onism (n.) - the frustration of being stuck in just one body, that inhabits only one place at a time, with the awareness of how little of the world you'll experience.

37. Opia (n.) - the intensity of looking someone in the eye, which can feel simultaneously invasive and vulnerable.

38. Rubatosis (n.) - the unsettling awareness of your own heart-beat.

39. Rückenfigur (n.) - the hypothetical view of the self from behind, retracing the path you took through the world.

40. Ruckkehrunruhe (n.) - the feeling of returning home after an immersive trip only to find it fading rapidly from your awareness.

41. Scintilla (n.) - a tiny, brilliant flash or spark that persists momentarily after ignition.

42. Semaphorism (n.) - a conversational hinted feeling that you have something personal to say on the subject but don't go any further.

43. Silience (n.) - the kind of unnoticed excellence that carries on around you every day.

44. Sonder (n.) - the realisation that each passerby has a life as complex as your own.

45. Sonderkommando (n.) - a person who is forced to do un-pleasant or dangerous tasks for someone else; especially in a Nazi death camp.

46. Sublimation (n.) - the transformation of unwanted impulses into something less harmful or even positive.

47. The Convolution of Fate (n.) - the process by which fate slips through your hands, as when you run into someone you were just thinking about or bump into a stranger who becomes a loved one.

48. The Vivisepulture (n.) - the horrifying realisation that you've been buried alive, and that not only is there no way out, but the air is already getting thin and your body is beginning to dehydrate and decompose, and eventually all you'll have left inside your coffin is your own despair and the growing hallucinations of your own doomed fantasies.

49. Theonoe (n.) - a divine presence that is felt but cannot be seen.

50. Tintinnabulation (n.) - the ringing or sound of bells.

51. Trenchant (adj.) - Keenly perceptive or sharp

52. Vagary (n.) - an unexpected and inexplicable change in a situation or someone's behaviour.

53. Vellichor (n.) - the strange wistfulness of used bookstores.

54. Vemödalen (n.) - the fear that everything has already been done.

55. Wytai (n.) - a feature of modern society that suddenly strikes you as absurd and grotesque – like the awareness that we slaughter animals for meat products

56. Xeno (n.) - the awareness of the smallest measurable unit of human connection, typically exchanged between passing strangers—flirtatious glances, warm smiles, sympathetic eyebrow raises—small fleeting moments and interactions that can alleviate the symptoms of feeling alone

57. Zenosyne (n.) - the sense that time keeps going faster and faster.

The subject of emotions, feelings, and their definitions seems to be inexhaustible, as each culture has added or subtracted from their vocabulary feeling states that resonate or no longer resonate with their overall experience at a societal level. As linguists have proven, the words we use are a mirror of our emotional life. Human beings have a need to put into words that which they experience, both to achieve a better understanding of themselves and to accurately communicate their reality to others. So, the more emotional depth we are capable of, the more words we create, and the more we get to experience and record "life".

From the number and diversity of terms presented above, which in no way represent a complete list of emotions and feeling states, we can conclude that the complexity of the IcNS is entirely required for dealing with the emotional complexity of human existence. As a human being, the experience of "life"- of being alive- can be only FELT – and that can be done only through emotions, feelings, and physical sensations. Without this "translation" of the outside into our inner universe – into our heart brain, we are faced with a sequence of events that we can logically understand – but that serve no purpose whatsoever.

OUR MAIN PURPOSE IN LIFE – RATIONALLY SPEAKING

In Dr. Herman Medow's book "Neuroplasticity. Biology of Psychotherapy" (2016), the brain goals have been identified as follows:

1. Surviving
2. Avoiding harm
3. Seeking pleasure

Combined, they lead to the following process of our rational mind:

Staying alive to be able to fulfill the goal of experiencing happiness in the safest way possible.

So, the main purpose in life- directed by our logical function itself- is to reach AN EMOTION. Because HAPPINESS IS AN EMOTION.

People who come into therapy are stuck in the first two phases and are seeking help to reach the third one.

No wonder we've yet to grasp the meaning of life. Have you noticed how happy people never ask this question? Because they know it- they can feel that everything is as it should be – the goal is reached. However, since the state of happiness is, by its own very emotional nature, temporary, this goal embedded in our brain ensures that we are never left without a purpose in life – and it becomes a perpetual reason to continue living.

So, happiness is much more than a desire, it's the direction our cognitive processes, beliefs, behaviours, coping mechanisms- are leading us towards, incessantly, until our brain activity stops. Our "hearts" take note of "where we are" relative to this goal and our "brains" direct us towards it. The human organism functions best when these two systems work together – and it experiences emotional, mental, and physical "malfunctions" – illnesses- when they work one against the other.

However, even if our logical brain makes all the "right" decisions towards us experiencing happiness, it must take into account the information received from the IcNS- as the system FEELS life, FEELS if the goal has been reached. As such, when there is information about emotional trauma in the system, it MUST find a way to either neutralise it or minimise it – to ensure the goal is still reachable. If we analyse every decision and every behaviour from this point of view, we can easily identify the ways in which the logical brain has attempted to do exactly that.

Unfortunately, we can't establish homeostasis in a pleasant emotional state if we are continuously "drowning" in unpleasant feelings triggered very easily. The painful emotional memories are still a reality even after we pushed them out of our conscientious awareness. And they will continuously be sent as information to the main brain – and be available for immediate reference when both nervous systems make use of their previously accumulated knowledge to analyse and understand current outside circumstances and events.

When an emotionally difficult experience is still present, recorded, and not completely archived, the awareness of the passing of time has no influence on those memories- they are still perceived as "open items". These high-intensity negative memories are like "clots" in the emotional pathways and the information of the activated emotional map is continuously sent to the main brain, causing ruminating thoughts, intrusive memories, etc. That is behind the mechanism of a trigger – and why the heart brain reaches those emotions so fast.

When they are activated- meaning triggered –it simply means that one element from that memory- any of the information recorded by the senses and the feelings that make up that specific memory (scents, words, colours, things, how people were "felt", their looks, environment, etc.) – has been found as already existing in the IcNS recorded memory. The entire outside reality will then be emotionally translated in the same way the initial experience was- as if it is a life experience from the same category- because we first FEEL life. We first learn how to emotionally "decode" life experiences, and, after we learned how- we decode them the same way.

The main brain will then access the actions it undertook related to that previous experience- and will provide the same directions- an irrational belief, a harmful behaviour or completely cutting off that event from rational awareness- whichever directive it considers would faster lead to survival, safety, and lastly, happiness.

Thus, in addition to properly completing the emotional integration of our real-time experiences, it is imperative, for the overall quality of our lives, to pay attention to and work on "de-clotting" our emotional pathways, in order to be able to sustain a pleasant emotional existence day in, day out. From this point of view, triggers are immensely helpful, as they indicate exactly where the problem lies- and they give us access to the memories, to be able to help the brain with the process of archiving them safely.

Here I have to mention that there is the highly disadvantageous belief that life should always be positive, that happiness, once reached, should last forever, and that problems arising in our life indicate that "we are not there yet". As mentioned above, all progress in life depends on the existence and overcoming of situations that get translated through not-so-pleasant emotions. **This is normal and necessary for the human life experience.**

Happiness is more like an all-encompassing emotional state, and it is the additional effect we get every time we reach one of the other desired emotions. However, it can also equate with a baseline of inner peace – which is reached when the amount of emotional trauma is minimal, the outside focus is positive, and the overall mindset is led by trust in one's own ability to deal with obstacles.

THE DIFFERENCE BETWEEN EMOTIONAL AND MENTAL ILLNESS

Emotional illness is the prolonged negative emotional state resulting from an emotional wound that has been left untreated for a certain amount of time and has accumulated high amounts of disturbing feelings from additional experiences that have had similar feeling signatures, overwhelming the emotional system and disrupting its overall activity.

Mental illness is the symptom of the existence of an emotional illness, where the mind's ability to function correctly has been impaired.

From a biological point of view, the number of neurons in the IcNS increased with every reiteration of that specific negative feeling signature, until, following its information transfer to the brain, it influenced the brain's activity- thoughts, beliefs, behaviours, coping mechanisms, to the point where it affected its overall capacity to function properly.

The relationship between emotional trauma and mental illness is a very simple one:

A distressed emotional system is AT THE ROOT of all mental illness.

In fact, what we call "mental illness" is nothing more but an accurate translation into thoughts, words, and coping mechanisms of a traumatised "emotional map of the world". In most cases, there is nothing wrong with the brain- unless it has severe fragmentation where parts leak into one another chaotically, or it has already advanced to physical brain damage. It just translates what it receives- and then directs its whole activity – the thoughts that affect the physical body included- from that emotional stand-point. The attempt to permanently change the thoughts without changing the emotional information the brain receives is logical to fail. So is the attempt to provide chemical adjuvants to promote different thoughts or feeling states- for the same reason. They may work temporarily- but they are not a permanent solution, unless we supply them to the body for the entire period of our life, which, then, defeats the purpose of both systems.

We can infer that the result of ongoing physical sensations kept alive by an untreated emotional trauma is the cause for certain physical illnesses- whose effect would decrease once the emotional component is neutralised.

The tranquillity of mind and certainty of moral worth thought by the stoic philosophy to be reachable only through complete rationality – is entirely possible and the worthiest endeavour. Once you are aware of your mental and behavioural activity derived as a response to an untreated emotional trauma, you can actually integrate the traumatised memory. Once you do so, there won't be any need to force yourself to be entirely rational against your feelings, as both systems will point in the same direction- the same choices, the most rational behaviours- in your best interest- to achieve safety and joy.

It is entirely possible to reach heart-driven decisions that make perfect sense.

AN INTEGRATIVE APPROACH TO HEALTH

On this note, we must also draw attention to the other scale of the balance – the danger of considering the heart brain "ruling" over the mind. That is incorrect and may lead to very poor decisions, as it all depends on the state of the established emotional map. If a person is carrying deep emotional wounds, listening only to their feelings and emotions will lead to behaviours designed to cope with them, instead of making the more rational decision of going against them for a better outcome, as they are not integrated and won't lead to a better quality of life.

As such, the process of healing requires paying attention to and addressing it on all of its 4 different levels:

1. Emotional circulation – being in the present moment, receiving and paying attention to all stimuli, and ensuring a complete emotional cycle through deep respiration , focus and acceptance of the perceived reality - **PRESENT**

2. Emotional integration – wounds healing/integrating childhood emotional trauma - **PAST**

3. Somatic healing – focusing on releasing the physical sensations recorded in the body during trauma and on creating new pleasant sensations to be recorded and remembered by the body – **PAST + FUTURE**

4. Mind-achieved health- identifying and changing assigned meanings from detrimental/that don't benefit us - to constructive/that benefit us, and an additional intentional focus on creating good-feeling thoughts – the voluntary and intentional creation of thoughts (through visualisation, positive focus, positive reminders and triggers, meditation, speech, etc.) that makes use of the mind, by enabling it to create

thoughts that, when transmitted to the heart, get translated into positive feelings (not only joy/happiness, but also the feeling of achievement, of pride in one's own work, the relief of making progress, and any other feeling that gets created following a process that needed to be recorded and analysed from a timeframe perspective). This ensures the creation of future healthy emotional states. It is also the process of intentional movement of one's own life towards a specific goal – **PRESENT+FUTURE**

IV

UNDERSTANDING HUMAN BEHAVIOUR

THE PYRAMID OF HUMAN NEEDS

In every ecosystem, the main function is that of the transfer of energy from one factor to another, in a cyclical manner, which ensures the achievement of balance. Balance is health.

The human body is, in fact, very similar to an ecosystem.

As in every ecosystem, the needs of the first functional factor are the primary needs of the system, the place where the cycle of energy transfer begins. When they are not fulfilled, the entire ecosystem is thrown out of balance- and becomes "ill", a chain reaction that affects it in its entirety.

The first functional system in the human body is the IcNS- the heart brain- with the affective function. From this, we can safely conclude that our emotional needs are our ecosystem's primary needs. Balance and health start from having them fulfilled.

Starting with 1943, Abraham Maslow and his colleague Carl Rogers (psychologists), have introduced the behavioural psychology theory, stating that people's actions are motivated by physiological and psychological needs, in a hierarchical order, from simple to complex.

However, their "Hierarchy of needs", which is the model that has been used until now, does not take into account the new scientifically proven neurobiological reality, as the information was not yet available at the time. As such, it must be re-arranged to mirror the discoveries of the 21st century. We will update the hierarchy by integrating into it the most current information available.

As per Maslow, there are 5 levels of needs:

1. Physiological Needs – they include those that are vital to survival (they mirror the brain's first goal – Survival). Food, water, air/breathing, shelter, sexual reproduction, homeostasis.
2. Security and Safety Needs – only concerning individuals that have their physiological needs met- they mirror the brain's second goal- Safety.

These first 2 needs groups are considered "basic needs" by Maslow and his colleague.

With the 3rd group, they begin talking about emotional needs such as:

1. The Social Needs – love, acceptance, belonging, etc;
2. Esteem Needs – appreciation, respect, self-esteem, personal worth;
3. Self-Actualisation Needs – the need to achieve their full potential.

However, we now know that the brain ensures survival and safety based on the emotional information received- the state of the emotional map. As such, that state will influence actions and behaviours, making the brain make "irrational" decisions toward survival, safety, and joy/pleasure.

Since the hierarchy of needs has been designed with the purpose of understanding what exactly drives human behaviour, and human behaviour is in response to thoughts that translate our emotions, then the basic needs are those of our emotional system.

As such, emotional needs that create the emotional map of the world that, then, becomes the blueprint for how the brain designs its own "map", are to be considered of primary importance.

Our emotional needs consist of nothing else but the need to experience healthy and pleasant emotions, after ensuring emotional survival and emotional safety.

Human beings are born with the intrinsic need of experiencing a vast diversity of positive emotions – the goal of "seeking pleasure" –, from which a select few are basic and universally required as lived experience. When the experience is denied, the child records, in turn, the negative emotion associated with the lack of fulfilment of a specific emotional need.

We can experience the following pleasant/healthy emotions (the list is far from complete):

LIST OF POSITIVE EMOTIONS

1. Admiration	20. Elation	38. Jubilation
2. Adoration	21. Emotional	39. Kindness
3. Aesthetic	connection	40. Life witnessing
Appreciation	22. Emotional	41. Longing
4. Affection	validation	42. Love
5. Amusement	23. Empathy	43. Lust
6. Arousal	24. Enchantment	44. Melancholy
7. Awe	25. Enthusiasm	45. Nostalgia
8. Belonging	26. Euphoria	46. Passion
9. Bliss	27. Excitement	47. Pleasure
10. Calm	28. Exhilaration	48. Pride
11. Care	29. Fascination	49. Relief
12. Cheerfulness	30. Friendship	50. Serenity
13. Compassion	31. Flirtation	51. Surprise
14. Contentment	32. Happiness	52. Sympathy
15. Curiosity	33. Hope	53. Tenderness
16. Delight	34. Interest	54. Triumph
17. Desire	35. Intrigue	55. Trust
18. Ease	36. Joviality	56. Uplift
19. Ecstasy	37. Joy	57. Wonder

There are 2 major ways in which emotional trauma arises:

- The majority of emotional trauma arises from those emotions that can be fulfilled only through others- in the context of relationships, such as: being/feeling loved, being treated with kindness, having justice, being treated with fairness, experiencing other people's empathy towards us, being protected (physical safety), being defended, being treated with care as to not be hurt (emotional safety), belonging (being accepted as part of a group), emotional connection (the different types of love: platonic, romantic, family), being admired, being treated with compassion, being trusted, having a trustworthy emotional connection (thus experiencing how it feels to trust others), truthful mirroring (emotional validation), life witnessing (companionship), etc.

- The rest occurs when a specific positive emotion is simply being denied - either directly or by being branded as "unacceptable"- curiosity, awe, pride, pleasure, passion, wonder, triumph, lust, flirtation, excitement, euphoria, arousal, ecstasy, delight, joviality, interest, happiness, etc.

How many of these are considered unsuitable or undesirable in children? And yet, we have to experience and record them by age 8-9 - if we want to be able to recognise them and re-create them in healthy ways later in life.

As a conclusion, the updated Pyramid of Human Needs—meaning the hierarchy in which human needs influence human decision-making and behaviours—is as follows:

1. Emotional Survival needs – assessed within the context of human relationships: emotional connection(closeness) and belonging;
2. Emotional Safety needs – assessed within the context of human relationships: emotional validation, fairness, kindness, trust, honesty, empathy, compassion, etc.;
3. Physical Survival and Safety needs: air, water, food, physical health; shelter, physical integrity, safe environment;

4. Intellectual Survival and Safety needs – the need for understanding, the need for clarity, the need for meaning congruence (the same situation/person must fit into the initially assigned meaning, to provide intellectual safety), the need for coherence (between the external reality and the emotional translation) the need for intellectual validation; the need for accumulation of knowledge in order to better understand and be better suited for solving life difficulties;

5. Emotional, intellectual, and physical needs that offer positive emotions. Their order of importance is positively correlated with individual personal values, which differ from person to person.

A different view of understanding human behaviour emerges when we arrange emotions in antonymic or contrasting pairs, highlighting the negative emotions that human beings are trying to avoid:

- Aesthetic Disapproval - Aesthetic Appreciation
- Agitation - Calmness
- Agony - Ecstasy
- Anger - Calmness
- Angst - Contentment
- Annoyance - Delight
- Anxiety – Relaxation/ Safety
- Apathy - Enthusiasm/ Empathy/ Interest/ Passion/ Curiosity
- Aversion - Affection/ Desire
- Bitterness - Sweetness
- Boredom - Stimulation/ Excitement/Amusement/ Interest/ Intrigue
- Confusion - Clarity

- Contempt - Respect
- Cruelty - Kindness
- Defeat - Victory
- Defiance - Compliance
- Depression - Euphoria
- Depression - Elation/Exhilaration/Contentment
- Despair - Hope
- Despondency - Glee
- Detestation - Adoration
- Disappointment - Satisfaction
- Disapproval - Admiration/Acceptance/Approval
- Disbelief - Belief
- Discontent - Contentment
- Disgust - Delight/Appreciation/ Lust
- Disinterest - Awe /Fascination/ Flirtation/ Interest
- Dismalness - Joviality
- Distrust - Trust
- Dread - Anticipation
- Disenchantment - Enchantment
- Embarrassment - Confidence
- Envy - Admiration
- Exhaustion - Rest
- Fear - Courage
- Frustration - Satisfaction
- Fury - Calmness
- Grief - Joy
- Guilt - Innocence
- Hatred/Fear/Aversion - Love
- Heartbreak - Healing
- Helplessness - Empowerment
- Horror - Delight
- Hostility - Friendliness

- Humiliation - Pride
- Hysteria - Composure
- Indifference - Compassion
- Indignation - Acceptance
- Insecurity - Confidence
- Insult - Compliment
- Irritation - Calmness
- Isolation - Inclusion
- Jealousy - Contentment
- Killing - Mercy
- Loathing - Love
- Loneliness – Friendship/Life witnessing
- Longing - Fulfilment
- Melancholy - Euphoria
- Misery - Happiness/ Bliss
- Morbidness - Cheerfulness
- Neglect - Care
- Nervousness - Calmness
- Nostalgia - Novelty
- Outrage - Approval
- Overwhelm - Underwhelm
- Panic - Calmness
- Rejection - Belonging
- Sadness - Happiness
- Sorrow - Joy

Just by a simple look, we can all agree that human beings are striving to run from, get rid of, or control negative emotions- and those considered as "negative" by the societal norms of the specific period in history.

However, from the point of interest of emotional trauma therapy, we must take into consideration the fact that the mechanism giving rise to these subjective sensations is mapped out in child-hood- we learn them from our environment and other people. As psychoanalyst D. W. Winnicott explains, "the Mirror Stage" in childhood development consists of a child internalising their mother's emotional reaction to them, reaction registered first from their mother's face. However, the child internalises ANY emotion that is shown- first from their mother, then their extended family environment, then the larger social environment. This is how the mechanism of giving rise to an emotion later in life is initially set up - we learn to feel specific emotions and feelings in specific cir-cumstances, and the knowledge adds up, solidifying the mechanism with a database of situations when the particular emotions are an appropriate translation (reaction) of life. And this knowledge is also very useful to the individual, as it assists with directing their life away from pain and towards good-feeling states.

When the child starts to learn language, it associates words with the specific emotions that have already been translated and recorded as feeling states and sensations in specific parts of the body. The language function comes as an addition, a link between the mental system and the emotional system. That is the reason why, later in life, people can experience feeling states and bodily sensations by making use of thoughts and words, as we are able to recreate them from the information recorded in our Intracardiac Nervous system, without the need for the specific circumstances to actually be happening in our outside reality.

The infant is looking for positive feeling states. The outside reality felt as a negative emotion is nothing more than the lack of fulfilment of an emotional need derived from this need for experi-encing positive emotions- in order to map them out and allow the brain to, later in life, fulfil its quest of seeking pleasure, survival, safety – of creating a life by providing the experiences the heart brain translates into emotions, so that we can feel that life. As we learn what life is and how it feels, we learn to decode feeling states-there is no other way to feel life, that is the beginning of the process, as indicated above. Thoughts, sensations, etc, are the "translation". Negative emotions are, thus, nothing more than the information that something necessary is missing, so we can use them as a driver for change and progress. This does not apply, though, to emotional trauma, which is an emotional overwhelm that blocks progress.

In the 2014 study "Bodily map of emotions", Dr. Glerean and his colleagues concluded that there must be a biological basis for the association between emotions and bodily sensations, as they proved to activate the same body areas, regardless of the specific culture of study participants. "Feelings, or fear, can be frozen so that we experience numbness instead of sensations," he says. "That is linked to shock, and as we start to heal, the shock melts and the underlying sensations do come to the surface."

WHEN WE FEEL EMOTIONS, WHERE DO THEY HAPPEN?

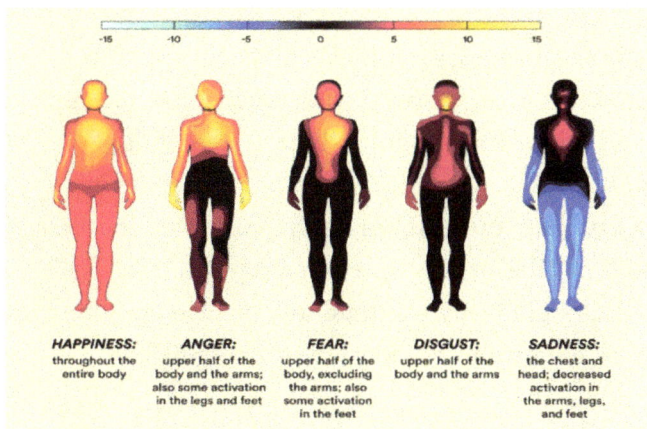

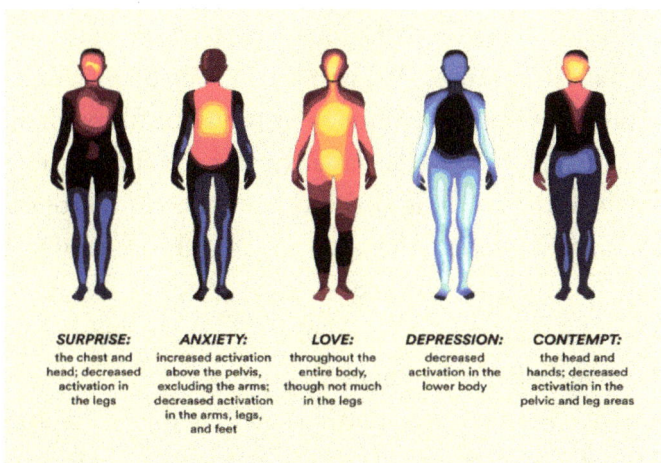

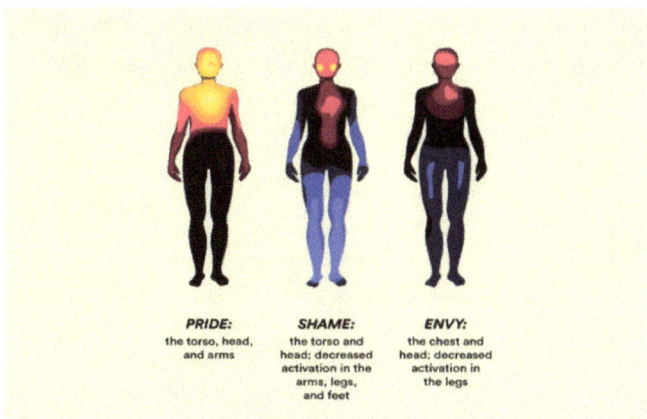

HAPPINESS:
throughout the
entire body

ANGER:
upper half of the
body and the arms;
also some activation
in the legs and feet

FEAR:
upper half of the
body, excluding
the arms; also
some activation
in the feet

DISGUST:
upper half of the
body and the arms

SADNESS:
the chest and
head; decreased
activation in
the arms, legs,
and feet

SURPRISE:
the chest and
head; decreased
activation in
the legs

ANXIETY:
increased activation
above the pelvis,
excluding the arms;
decreased activation
in the arms, legs,
and feet

LOVE:
throughout the
entire body,
though not much
in the legs

DEPRESSION:
decreased
activation in the
lower body

CONTEMPT:
the head and
hands; decreased
activation in the
pelvic and leg areas

PRIDE:
the torso, head,
and arms

SHAME:
the torso and
head; decreased
activation in the
arms, legs,
and feet

ENVY:
the chest and
head; decreased
activation in
the legs

https://greatist.com/connect/emotional-body-maps-infographic#
infographic

In the above images, increased activity corresponds with warmer colours (red, orange, yellow), while decreased/ lacking responses correspond with cooler colours (blue, green, indigo, black) as if it were a heat map.

If we consider the emotion of happiness as the basic primary translation of "life", then we can extrapolate that the areas with cooler colours gradually translate less intense emotions until they show up as either non-responsive or overwhelmed with negative input.

We are meant to interact with our environment with our entire body- through our senses. When parts of our body are shown as not "activated" by certain emotions, it translates through a lack of interaction between our external environment and ourselves. We are rejecting acknowledging the information coming from outside, we don't want to accept the external stimuli, there is a lack of emotional information in that body area, a "lack of life", if you will. We are not functioning as we should. The areas that are activated mark the areas where the chemical components of the associated emotions have been released and the associated physical sensations are allowed to be felt. However, the fact that the areas that have not been activated are shown as dark in the above images highlights the lack of any physical sensation- so, either partial release of hormones and neuropeptides or an overwhelm.

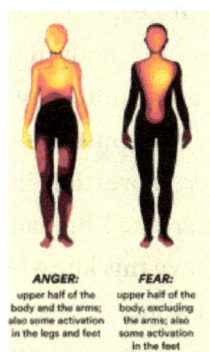

ANGER:
upper half of the
body and the arms;
also some activation
in the legs and feet

FEAR:
upper half of the
body, excluding
the arms; also
some activation
in the feet

greatist.com/connect/
emotional-body-maps
-infographic

For example, when we feel intense fear, we can all attest that our legs go numb, to the point that, sometimes, we cannot move them.

In prolonged anger, our lower abdomen/stomach starts hurting – indicating that it has been experiencing overwhelming muscle contractions that we were not aware of.

As such, the physical component of the emotional wounds that are not fully processed are indicated by the dark areas in the study images. What is healthy is to have the entire body respond- more or less- to an external event. When there are non-responsive areas, that is an indication of the existence of a refusal to physically feel the associated sensations, that would enable the emotional circulation to be successful and complete. During the emotional integration of a painful memory, we are simply allowing the stacked-up chemicals to be released and fully felt in their respective body areas, which leads to the body being able to restore its proper functioning, without the constant chemical (emotional) overwhelm.

If we want to modify the recorded information in the "emotional map of the world", when reaching any traumatic memory, we must ensure that, after we allow the feeling to complete its cycle, we create in our imagination a reality that would be translated through the positive emotions and more complex emotional needs that were missing in the initial experience. This imagined reality must be sustained until it is felt as feelings and sensations in the body, informing us that the mapped information has been updated.[1]

The study participants were chosen from different geographical regions, speaking their native languages. However, the body topography they indicated for each emotion showed great similarity, regardless of the country differences, which leads to the conclusion that emotions have a fixed pre-determined sensory expression in the human body – which makes it a feature of generalised human anatomy. Further on, this indicates that our bodies have this knowledge embedded before socialisation (which is country-specific)- e.g. we are born with the directive of where in our body each emotion is felt (which body area must be activated by each emotion)- before our brains are developed.

The below Emotional Guidance Scale assists us greatly in identifying the emotional hierarchy per intensity/de-activation felt in the body:

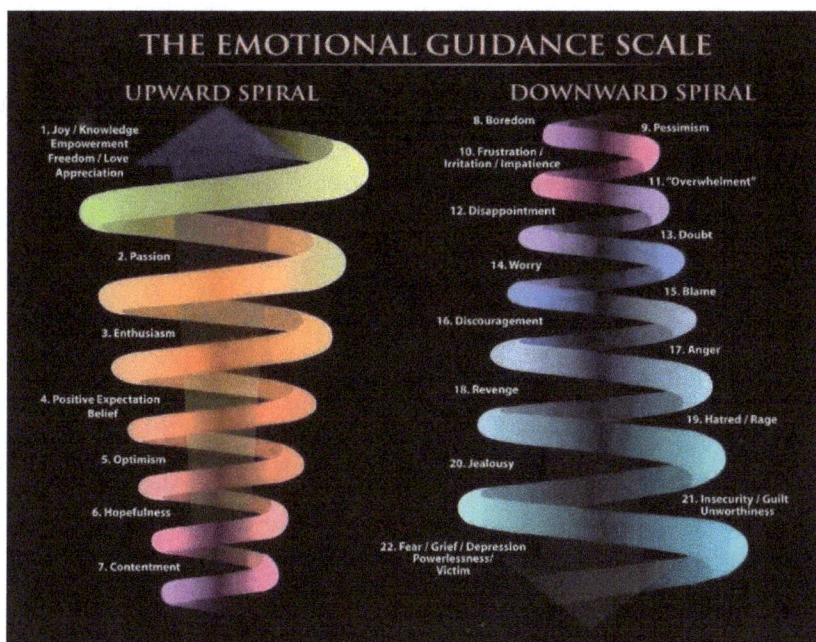

THE EMOTIONAL GUIDANCE SCALE

UPWARD SPIRAL — DOWNWARD SPIRAL

1. Joy / Knowledge / Empowerment / Freedom / Love / Appreciation
2. Passion
3. Enthusiasm
4. Positive Expectation / Belief
5. Optimism
6. Hopefulness
7. Contentment
8. Boredom
9. Pessimism
10. Frustration / Irritation / Impatience
11. "Overwhelment"
12. Disappointment
13. Doubt
14. Worry
15. Blame
16. Discouragement
17. Anger
18. Revenge
19. Hatred / Rage
20. Jealousy
21. Insecurity / Guilt / Unworthiness
22. Fear / Grief / Depression / Powerlessness / Victim

in5d.com/the-emotional-guidance-scale/

COVER EMOTIONS

In order to protect against very low de-activation (with its corresponding intracardiac brainwave frequency carried by the specific feeling), the emotional system has a fail-safe mechanism in place: the "cover" emotions. These are the emotions at the base of the downward spiral, which can be very dangerous to the body if experienced for too long. When they are part of an emotional reality that keeps being re-activated, their feeling signatures will be covered by higher, more body-activating emotions. In this category, we have:

- Anger – gets the system out of extreme and prolonged fear;
- Hatred – gets the system out of extreme and prolonged emotional hurt/pain;
- Numbness – covers shock or confusion;
- Desperation – keeps the person out of despair.

MIXED FEELINGS

Although some of the emotions are just different degrees of the same emotional state, either positive or negative, we often experience what we call "mixed feelings", a mixture of positive and negative feelings arising from the same external situation, producing confusion and usually resulting in an inability to make a decision and/or act on it. The "mixed feelings" situation is related to the existence of different "parts/voices" within our psyche, that translate the experience in accordance with their own pre-established set of beliefs and their own emotional needs, drawing their own conclusions relative to what would benefit them most, which can be different or even oppositional in actual behavioural commands from the initial decision - hence, giving rise to a resistance to act.

This can be easily identified in the "habit" of procrastination. The individual might say and be convinced that they want to perform a specific task, however, they can't "make themselves" accomplish or even start it. In therapy, there is an investigation into the reasons for every part/voice involved, and decisions are made in accordance with the specific personal truth revealed and with the cooperation of both "parts/voices".

IRRATIONAL BELIEFS IN ADULTHOOD

Irrational beliefs are a series of fixed thinking patterns that take into account a very limited view of reality, with no room for healthy adaptive strategies. When these beliefs have been adopted as personal values, people judge and analyse life experiences, make decisions, and adopt behaviours that prove to be harmful towards themselves, others, or society at large, in the long run. Their purpose is that of keeping the individual safe from experiencing certain negative feelings that are perceived to be unavoidable should the fixed requirement be unfulfilled. They represent nothing more but the brain performing its main task- that of keeping the individual safe – this time, from negative emotions.

Below is a list of some of the irrational beliefs commonly identified in adults:

- I absolutely MUST succeed in everything I do OTHERWISE I am a worthless person (*I will feel unimportant/inferior/weak*).
- I absolutely MUST succeed in everything I do OTHERWISE it's terrible and catastrophic for me (it's the worst thing that could happen to me – *I will feel immense suffering*).
- I absolutely MUST succeed in everything I do OTHERWISE I cannot tolerate/endure it (it is unbearable for me – *I will experience a very unpleasant, painful, and upsetting feeling*).
- It is IMPERATIVE that others treat me properly and/or nicely OTHERWISE it is definitive proof that I am worthless as a person (*I will feel unimportant/inferior/weak*).
- It is IMPERATIVE that others treat me properly and/or nicely OTHERWISE it's terrible and catastrophic for me (it's the worst thing that could happen to me - *I will feel immense suffering*).

- It is IMPERATIVE that others behave correctly and/or nicely towards me OTHERWISE I cannot tolerate/endure it (It is unbearable for me - *I will experience a very unpleasant, painful, and upsetting feeling*).
- It is IMPERATIVE that others behave correctly and/or nicely OTHERWISE it is definitive proof that they are wrong, evil, rotten individuals (*I will feel betrayed, disgusted, unsafe*).
- Life SHOULD always be fair, and life SHOULD always be easy OTHERWISE it is definitive proof that life is bad, and *I will always be in pain.*
- Life SHOULD always be fair, and life SHOULD always be easy OTHERWISE it's terrible and catastrophic for me (it's the worst thing that could happen to me - *I will feel immense suffering*).
- Life SHOULD always be fair, and life SHOULD always be easy OTHERWISE I can't tolerate it (it's unbearable for me - *I will experience a very unpleasant, painful, and upsetting feeling*).
- I MUST be liked by everyone around me OTHERWISE it is definitive proof that I am worthless as a person/ it's terrible and catastrophic for me/ I can't tolerate it (*I will feel worthless/ immense suffering/ a very unpleasant, painful, and upsetting feeling that I won't be able to endure*).
- MYSELF, OTHERS AND/OR LIFE SHOULD ALWAYS... OTHERWISE, *I will suffer.*

These beliefs are considered to be "irrational" when held by adults. However, we must remember that they have been adopted following repeated experiences encountered in childhood – and so, they are the result of an attempt at safety performed by an insufficiently developed brain, along with the child actually being in a very difficult situation where there weren't many other options available.

The child is, indeed, in the impossibility of removing themselves from the experiences or circumstances that cause them pain but are performed by their family.

Thus, when living with a highly demanding, criticising, or downright narcissistic parent, it is extremely important- a MUST – to be perfect, to ensure you are liked, to ensure you keep them to a high standard of goodness and fairness, otherwise they might hurt you with their "evil" behaviour, and so on. These beliefs are no longer irrational when we understand that they are coping mechanisms that served a very specific purpose – that of keeping the child safe from re-experiencing emotional, mental, and, possibly, physical trauma.

The adults who still carry these fixed thinking patterns do not have mental health issues- their brain functions perfectly. What they have is emotional trauma that needs to be listened to and integrated.

Since they have these emotional wounds, they still get re-actualised and the adult indeed feels the associated pain every time that specific situation is repeated, e.g. when someone around them displays a behaviour that highlights that they are not liked, the adult feels the initial pain of rejection and the fear of emotional unsafety that they felt in their childhood. So, from this point of view, the "irrational" belief still keeps them safe from pain- at least in that specific situation. Of course, if still held in adulthood, these beliefs cause pain in other areas of life, but, since they still fulfil their initial purpose, the brain will choose to keep them until it is given a more viable and safer alternative.

After the initial emotional wound is addressed and the parts of the psyche storing it are made aware of the new reality- that the danger of experiencing the same pain is greatly reduced, the brain will naturally let go of these coping mechanisms, replacing them with others that will continue to keep the individual safe in the newly-observed life circumstances. As a result, the related coping behaviours will be adjusted, as well.

[1]A complete guide on how to achieve this on your own can be found in the book "The Completion Process" by Teal Swan.

V

PRIMARY EMOTIONAL NEEDS

THE NEED FOR CONNECTION/CLOSENESS

The need for emotional connection is the first and most important human need. In fact, we are born with this feeling already recorded and mapped, as we first experience it in uterus, along with feeling safe, belonging and love. Being so basic, it is mostly overlooked in children, as it is assumed that parents automatically form an emotional connection with their child, thus not being necessary to pay attention to its continuous fulfilment.

However, the reality is that, even though the child is perfectly able and eager and ready to preserve this primary connection, many adults are simply incapable of fully forming or maintaining this emotional connection. This is due to the following reasons:

1. parents don't know that, to raise a happy and healthy child, it is required to carefully maintain this connection at all times

through physical touch, empathy, kindness, compassion, acceptance, emotional validation, understanding and respect for the child's personal needs, desires, preferences, thoughts, feelings ("personal boundaries")

2. previously encountered emotional trauma that has caused the parents to reject deep emotional connection as a protection mechanism from emotional pain. They, themselves, are usually unaware of it, but the child feels that something is missing- as the child's emotional capacity to love, mirror and connect is at its highest. This faulty emotional connection mechanism from parents is what allows them to not be attuned to their child's emotional reality- and use punishment and criticism as an educational adjuvant or showing indifference to their child's emotional needs or blatantly contradicting a child's emotional needs in order to fulfil their own.

3. the method through which we currently carry out the process of socialisation – by placing social conformity above emotional health and diversity. This stems from the reality that, currently, due to a lack of knowledge and understanding, emotions are perceived as of a lower importance and a hindrance to education. This method creates immense amounts of emotional trauma, it cripples children's heart brain, and, through it, it becomes the number one reason for emotionally induced illnesses later in life.

An example of an emotionally traumatising event raised by an interruption of the parent-child emotional connection would be the moment when a child realises that the parent does not care that the child feels emotional pain following the parent's behaviour or words. During emotional trauma integration therapy, it has been noticed that the disconnection is physically experienced as deep muffled pain along all the veins and arteries in the body. Left untreated, it may lead to serious health issues within the circulatory system.

Initially, the child will choose to forget the event altogether, as it is an obstacle to experiencing the rest of the positive emotions that depend on the existence of a healthy emotional connection with the parent- belonging, trust, safety, etc. But its effects will not disappear just because the child pushed the awareness of it in the subconscious. That initial trauma becomes a "collection point" for all the following instances where they feel an emotional disconnection. Now, depending on how the child decides to "cope" to ensure that they won't experience the pain of disconnection again, we witness the adoption of one of the following dysfunctional attachment styles in relationships:

1. avoidant (becomes "dismissive" in adulthood),
2. anxious (becomes "preoccupied" in adulthood) and
3. disorganised (becomes "preoccupied-avoidant" in adulthood).

There are many other variations of coping mechanisms adopted as relationship styles, but, for the moment, we will discuss the main three presented above.

Society praising the self-sufficiency of autonomy does nothing more but voice one of the coping mechanisms we found in answer to this pain of disconnection – to avoid the pain of loneliness, betrayal, disappointment, find happiness within yourself, depend only on yourself, don't rely on others, be independent to the extreme- so, stay safe from experiencing pain when you lose the basic need of emotional connection. It is the belief adopted as a coping mechanism: "If you want to not suffer when it's gone, don't have it at all." This is completely unhealthy and AGAINST our own anatomy. It is a coping mechanism.

AVOIDANT ATTACHMENT STYLE

It is the result of the emotional trauma of enmeshment. The person has a deep need for connection, but they feel "claustrophobic" in a close relationship, as they invariably feel pushed to become a "copy" of the other person, forced to give up on their own individuality, in danger of "being controlled". As they have decided to identify with the "independent, self-reliant" personality, they perceive other people's requests as threats to their own sense of identity.

How does enmeshment present itself in a family setting?

The primary figure does not consider the child as an independent, individual entity, with their own autonomous self, but as a continuation of themselves, who is forced to want, need, perceive and choose to do only what the primary figure decides is best. There is no space for individuality- for personal feelings, personal thoughts, wishes, needs, desires- e.g. to have their own preferences, to choose their own clothes, friends, hobbies or career, etc. They are not allowed to conscientiously form an ego based on their own preferences. When they declare: "no, I don't want that, I want the other thing/something else.", they are met with painful consequences- either punishment or emotional abandonment. The child learns that other people will try and impose their own will at all costs – and that, choosing to be in a close relationship with them means choosing to be forced to comply and lose their individuality.

Thus, they are not aware of the possibility that someone else might actually care about their needs and desires.

However irrational it may be, this conclusion is entirely valid and understandable for them, even in adulthood, as the individual has never experienced the opposite in childhood. The imprinted experience is – "Because I loved them, I was obligated to do what they wanted and become what they liked, which brought me pain", -feeling forced to give up on their own needs, desires, preferences, thoughts, feelings, in order to preserve the emotional connection/ closeness/belonging and avoid the pain of disconnection/emotional abandonment. Thus, as a coping mechanism protecting them from the possibility of feeling that pain again, they have decided that they won't succumb to other people's emotional pressure anymore, ever. This gives them a feeling of control and personal power.

Society must be made aware of the fact that children must be allowed to correctly calibrate their own emotional system, which will be their guidance system towards good-feeling emotions and the fulfilment of their emotional needs their entire life.

However, when the parents interfere (as their desire is to have a well-behaved child, who listens to them and doesn't cause them any additional stress), the entire process is truncated, and the child goes through what is called "developmental trauma", where basic emotional needs remain unfulfilled. In essence, the child is not allowed to emotionally develop as they should to be able to create healthy beliefs and adopt socially healthy behaviours later in life. They are in effect forced to disregard what they really feel, need, think or want in order to not upset the parents and lose the sense of emotional connection and belonging within the family. Not following their internal "compass" obviously doesn't feel good, yet children so traumatised learn that this is a requirement for being in a relationship, and they will have the same felt experience in subsequent romantic (and not only) relationships - upon entering in a relationship, they will start feeling "controlled", as if the other person is trying to push onto them their own beliefs, behaviours, hobbies. The "avoidant" personality is trapped between needing to fulfil their basic human need for emotional connection and being in pain when trying to fulfil it in a relationship with another person.

In most cases, they have a very hard time identifying what they really like and what is their true character, as they were not allowed to develop a "core" – a strong and healthy ego – when they were children. By being told that "it is for their own good" as "parents know best", they have foregone their sense of knowing what feels good based on their own internal guidance, and they immediately adopt other people's "guidance", without even being asked to do so. As such, they will gravitate towards seemingly strong-willed individuals, who will either make up for their own lack of defined self (personal "boundaries" created by what they want and need, like and dislike, etc) or provide a strong definition that they can use as a point of reference to define themselves **against.**

In consequence, in adulthood, they will be in a continuous struggle to feel "defined", leaning towards being completely independent, unaware of their innate fear of relationships, being very "stubborn" in what they want. When they have adopted the coping mechanism of an avoidant style of relating, they will be incapable of finding "a middle ground" solution in conflict, as taking into consideration the partner's needs and feelings will feel like "losing" and a re-enactment of their childhood trauma. As such, they seem very self-absorbed and to value independence, when, in fact, they are just trying very hard to not "lose themselves" in the relationship. No matter how validating of their partner's needs they may seem and however careful they may explain to the partner their own needs, they will still be, in the end, dismissive of the other individual's feelings and needs, considering their own as more important – since the opposite would cause them pain and fear. The possibility of finding a third option that would satisfy both does not even occur to the avoidant individual, as they have not experienced it in childhood. They have never experienced a primary relationship where their best interests were taken into account when making a decision that would impact both, so they are unaware that another person may genuinely care about what feels good for them, as well. Every interaction with conflicting needs is experienced as a "passive war", the available choice is always only "either-or".

To change this dysfunctional style of relating, the person has to:

1. The first step- heal their enmeshment trauma by working to correctly calibrate their own emotional system (what should have happened in childhood). In order to accomplish that, the individual has to experience and record the feeling of freedom to choose what they really want, without any painful consequences in their relationships.

2. The second step, after learning that they are important, is to learn that both members in a relationship matter, so they must also become aware and experience how it feels to not only be impacted but also have an emotional impact on the other person – and learn how to look for and find the middle ground that best benefits both.

3. Experience, notice and record the feeling of deeper connection, happiness and harmony as a result of finding a middle ground that benefits both. Feeling safe in the relationship.

ANXIOUS ATTACHMENT STYLE

It is a result of the emotional trauma of abandonment.

We are born within the context of emotional connection – this need is not something to learn or experience in order to have it mapped (imprinted), as it is the initial basis of our experience after birth. The phase of individualisation is when the child gets imprinted with the rest of the emotional map, thus becoming a separate individual, with personal distinct traits that will dictate the experiences their brain will direct them to have in order to fulfil the rest of the available positive emotions during their own lifetime.

When the child could not conform to what the parents wanted (the request might also have been indirect or not voiced at all, but implied), the parents simply emotionally abandoned the child, creating the imprint of unpredictable pain in relationships- the pain and fear of loneliness that comes with the inevitability of being abandoned. This can be as simple as giving a child time-out for doing something the parent disliked, such as: sending them to stay in the corner or to their room, withholding normal conversation/ interaction to highlight parent disapproval, ignoring them as punishment, leaving home without them after chastising them, blaming and staying upset with them to make them remember that what they have done is not acceptable, etc. The child learns that the connection is not secure, and they cannot predict when they will feel the pain of disconnection again. To protect themselves from being abandoned, they adopt the coping mechanism of "holding tightly" to the parent. The emotional system is imprinted with the experience "I am not important to them", "I fear that they won't love me anymore", "I need them; they don't need me", "Loneliness is as painful as dying", "I'm in danger of losing them at any moment".

However, on top of those negative imprints, there is also the following limitation created as an effect of our current social structure: "There is no one else to love me, they are my whole family. If they don't love me, I am left completely alone – I am left to die." Due to the limited family resources present in day-to-day life (only the parents and, sometimes, one or two grandparents), children who are emotionally abandoned by one or both of their parents learn that love is scarce and that there is no one else who can accept them as an important and valuable part of the family.

In adulthood, they will feel a very strong need for close relationships, coupled with a very strong fear of losing the connection after it has been established. Through this fear, they will be completely at the mercy of the other person in the relationship, being unaware of their own value for the other person, and constantly needing reassurance that they are still loved. Their biggest fear is that of loneliness- resembling fear of death. They have learned in childhood that people's feelings are not to be trusted and that what they themselves feel doesn't matter so much to the other person. They feel a deep sense of being abandoned (and loneliness) and they carry that pain, along with the fear of re-experiencing it, their entire life. Every relationship is filtered through the frightening possibility of being abandoned again, without being able to pinpoint a rational reason for it, so without the possibility of ever finding how exactly to be and behave to ensure that the emotional connection is sound and safe and that their basic need is assured to be fulfilled. All they want and need is to be able to calm down their system with a sense of emotional safety.

In order to change this coping mechanism of feeling constant abandonment anxiety, the person has to undertake the following therapeutic steps:

1. Integrate the emotions of fear of abandonment, betrayal, rejection, loss of belonging, re-mapping the emotional map with the experience of an ever-lasting, loving and safe family environment.
2. Re-create the opposite experience in real-life connections– when getting anxious, the other person should be coming towards them, not away, making the connection more emotionally secure. For this, the partner must be made aware

of the pattern and must cooperate in creating a tight safe emotional environment when the anxiety is triggered.

3. Identify and integrate parts of the psyche that perpetuate the belief that the person is not valuable/important enough;

4. Increase the person's self-esteem through daily exercises and real-life experiences.

Since the heart brain continuously sends the information with the recorded emotional map and the emotional wounds to the main brain – whose job is to find solutions to diminish the pain and fulfil the missing emotional needs - **people with an anxious attachment style will unconsciously perceive the avoidant relationship style as "familiar", and vice-versa, and will enter into relationships with adults displaying that potential.** The hidden purpose is to finally heal the wounds and fulfil the needs. However, the other person has the exact opposite behaviour than what they really need, so they find themselves in the same pain they experienced in childhood – which can be used by both partners to identify their respective emotional wounds and integrate them.

DISORGANISED ATTACHMENT STYLE

This style of adapting is simply Stockholm Syndrome developed in a family setting.

We, as a society, are reluctant to take a deep analytical look at the emotional reality within a family environment, simply because we feel overwhelmed by the task. How can we, with the current social structure, be mindful of this, with people's emotional nature being so elusive?

And yet, this pattern is much more common than we care to admit.

Social carers and the other organisations that are striving to ensure children's safety are doing their best and we, as a society, owe them our gratitude. Their hard and dedicated work has positively impacted the lives of hundreds of millions of children.

However, when it comes to the disorganised attachment style, it is extremely difficult to identify how unstable and unpredictable the emotional reality is, just by looking at the child.

The mechanism behind it is the following: **"I am afraid, and I don't want to be near that person-** who hurts me, even if they are my parent- **but I can't escape, there is nowhere to go and no one else to love me,** because this is my home, my family, my life. So, I will pretend to comply – I will make them believe I am on their side, I will say, do and be exactly what they want me to be **so that I can avoid danger from their anger and still have a parent who cares for me." "I have to be friends with them, even if I am afraid of them or I don't like them." "I have to give them what they need- approval, love, admiration, loyalty- to ensure that they are not upset with me, and they don't abandon me or hurt me. However, I am pretending, this is not me- I have to get away from them to be <the real me>."**

From the outside, it is extremely easy to mistake this coping mechanism with being the child who has a very close and strong relationship with the parent who has all the power in the family- who is, also, the most overtly dangerous.

What the others don't see is the extreme fear the child feels, the feelings of betrayal and anger(the parent should have been the one to love them, not put them in danger), the extreme feeling of powerlessness (they can't leave and the other parent is weak, they cannot help them, as they themselves are under the control of the one with all the power), the deep feeling of loneliness and being forsaken (they are alone in this "emotional hell" and no one sees their pain), and, very often, an exacerbated need to protect the weaker parent and the other siblings.

This is the Disorganised Attachment style- a very strong bond built on fear. **Survival is ensured by being the abuser's best friend.**

When the abusive parent's behaviour is very unpredictable, children have to become proficient at "reading the room" – attuning to the parent's emotional state to know, in every second, how to respond when the abuser enters into one of their dangerous "parts" and how to de-escalate their negative emotions (how to make them feel better). In some cases, the child who manages to reach this high level of emotional attunement becomes the abusive parent's "favourite child" and, often, the child hated (envied) by all the other siblings (even if very well hidden, the child will feel it, as they learned how to attune to other people's feelings). This further isolates the child emotionally - a very confusing, painful and lonely situation which later may push the child towards the coping mechanism of suicide ideation.

In adulthood, this person will get very quickly attached, and then, will be terrified of both losing their own identity in the relationship - and of upsetting the partner and being abandoned. They will feel visceral fear, but they will be unable to explain it. They will become what the other person shows them they like and appreciate in a person, but they will (consciously or unconsciously) resent them for causing them to change. Even the slightest of criticisms will hurt immensely, as it will be translated with the meaning: "They don't like that"- which they learned is very dangerous.

On the one hand, they will do everything in their power to "keep the peace", keep the other person happy and content, be "good" and "endure", so as to not be abandoned, they will demand a very tight relationship, where the partners do everything together, praise, admiration, tokens of love. On the other hand, when hurt, they will feel a strong desire to leave the relationship immediately, so they may exert anger, accusations, even violent behaviour- the result of the very deep emotional pain triggered by the partner's behaviour.

As indicated above, they will enter into relationships with adults that display the potential for the same relationship style they learned in childhood- meaning- highly unpredictable, emotionally, psychologically and/or physically abusive. When their wounds are triggered, they will not react only to the partner's behaviour- they will react to ALL THE ABUSE they've been put through in their childhood – but their partner will seem as unresponsive to their requests as the parents were.

The adult with the disorganised attachment style will always want and dream of leaving the relationship, but they will find it emotionally impossible- and they will not understand the reason. They will be convinced that they must deeply love the person who is hurting them – because they are terrified of losing the partner, even when the partner displays intermittent abusive behaviour.

They will continuously be torn between the parts who want to leave (who keep reminding them of all of the hurt and suffering they went through in the relationship, the one who doesn't really want to be in any relationship, the one who has wanted to escape the childhood family environment, but was unable to, so it still wants to), and the parts who want to preserve the connection at all costs (who are convinced that leaving equates with death, the one that is consumed by fear of losing the feeling of belonging, the one that believes that this relationship is the only one available, the ones who feel unseen/unheard and need to be finally validated, and the ones that still keep all the other beliefs that were TRUE in their childhood, through a child's perception of life and available options.)

The difference between this type of relating and the previous two is the deep bond that is created and maintained through continuous cycles of abuse- love, pain-happiness, disappointment -hope, emotional detachment-emotional presence. **This is the process of trauma-bonding.**

The impression that the birth family relationship is strong will, usually, be preserved even years after leaving the family environment. Upon the abusive parent's death, the person with trauma-bond issues may experience an extremely painful re-owning of distressing memories that have been repressed for years, as the child needed to be able to keep the connection at all costs, and the memories were an obstacle. Now, the system feels it is safe to start the healing process- and it allows the person to access the pain that needs to be integrated. This may cause a brusque and seemingly overwhelming emergence of different negative emotional and mental states- from severe social anxiety to thoughts of being attacked or of being unable to survive.

THE NEED FOR APPROVAL

As we have established by now, the proper development of the heart brain in childhood drives us towards looking to record as many and as diverse "good feeling" experiences as possible. The need for approval is ensuring that we are going towards experiences that provide the knowledge of intimacy and closeness- feeling seen, heard and understood.

In cases where, in adulthood, there is an imbalanced need for approval, it can be traced back to having experienced chronic disapproval and criticism in childhood. Most likely, these two practices were used as "emotional blackmail" to force the child into submission and conformity- "to do as they're told", to accept the choices already made for them by their parents (and/or other siblings), regardless of their own desires.

Depending on the coping mechanism the child developed, we have two types of a dysfunctional need for approval in adulthood:

1. A **desperate need** for approval – the hallmark of the "golden child". In this case, the underlying feeling is that of **deep fear**, as the trauma is the loss of intimacy and closeness as a result of not conforming. This presupposes the initial successful fulfilment of this need – the child has first experienced approval several times, and the emotional memory has been successfully mapped. When met with disapproval and criticism, the child experienced a loss of intimacy and closeness. In order to keep themselves safe from re-experiencing the negative feeling of loss, the brain has chosen the coping mechanism of **conformity**. In adulthood, there is a desperate need for total approval, as lack of approval triggers the trauma of having lost intimacy, and the adult is deeply fearful of re-experiencing it. This trauma is one of the root causes of Shame and the "irrational" thinking patterns: "I absolutely MUST be perfect in everything I do/must succeed in everything" and "I absolutely MUST be liked by everyone." Also, the adult's reaction to constant criticism will be either

anxiety or its cover emotion, **anger**. This does not exclude the impact of Shame, which is the pain of deep loneliness.

2. A **very strong desire** for approval – the hallmark of the "scapegoated child". In this situation, whatever the child tried, it did not provide them with the experience of intimacy and closeness. The recorded emotional information is that of **deep pain**, the trauma is the pain of rejection, the complete refusal of emotional closeness in the family setting. Since we have these basic emotional needs throughout our entire lifetime (not only in childhood), in adulthood, the scapegoated child will have an exacerbated desire to experience the missing long-due positive feelings/emotions, which will make them feel accepted, seen, heard, understood. This trauma comes with the "irrational" thinking patterns: "It is IMPERATIVE that others treat me properly and/or nicely", "Life SHOULD always be fair, and life SHOULD always be easy". The adult's reaction to constant criticism (experienced as rejection) will be **deep emotional pain** (bordering on **despair**), with its cover emotion **Hate**. This does not exclude the anger resulting from the need for justice.

Even if the "golden child" carries Fear as the main driver, while the "scapegoated" one carries emotional Pain, the recorded emotional traumas are the same- the lack of closeness, intimacy, acceptance, belonging.

Once the root causes for the anxiety/anger/emotional pain/hate resulting from disapproval and criticism have been addressed, the emotional response in adulthood is greatly lowered in intensity.

THE NEED FOR JUSTICE

This is one of the most unaccepted emotional needs, not only in adults, but more so in children. It stems from the natural biological expectation, in childhood, that we should be loved, respected, seen, appreciated, and treated fairly in our family of origin. We expect friends and family to treat us as a friend and a family member. When these expectations are not met, we experience the feeling of betrayal- which is closely linked to injustice and unfairness. The betrayal trauma gives rise to resentment, anger and the desire for revenge. No matter how negatively portrayed these emotions are in current literature, they are still valid reactions to deep pain. The feeling of betrayal is one of the most painful experiences in one's life. When a child is being disrespected multiple times, their voice unheard, their preferences dismissed, their personal talents, inclinations and abilities unappreciated or criticised, they experience a feeling of betrayal, as there is an innate expectation of love, fairness and morality from the world, which is being broken. In consequence, children, as well as adults, become angry – which is entirely normal, valid and healthy. Their emotional reactions inform them that there is something happening that they don't like – **urging them to understand that unpleasant experience and change it.**

Without these emotions, we would never know when our environment is toxic for us and when we should strive to improve a situation.

Of course, parents do not like it when children display angry behaviour, so they, themselves, get angry at the child's emotion- as that emotion bothers them. It is very often that parents are bothered by their children's negative emotions, as they don't see the child as a functional human being yet, but as something to be moulded and taught how to behave "properly" – and a display of negative emotions might mean that they are failing at parenting. Moreover, parents must have immense amounts of patience and deep knowledge about their own emotions – in order to understand and feel at ease with another human being's emotions, a human being that is just learning about them and needs emotional guidance. Since most of us have denied our negative emotions in an attempt to feel better in our lives, it is highly uncomfortable for us when children naturally experience the valid translation of external events- e.g. they want a toy which they cannot have, so they get angry. If this experience gets repeated many times, the child will experience resentment at the unfairness of the situation- as well as the feeling of powerlessness- which they will carry on in adulthood.

The need for justice is recognised in situations of mental rumination – the constant repeating of certain situations in our mind, with made-up scenarios in which we defend ourselves, we say the right thing, we take the wanted action, in order to feel better prepared if it happens again. Or, in its passive state – a defeated attitude of cynicism, a total lack of hope of improvement and a negative view of people in general.

When justice is refused, the pain can trap a person in a thought pattern of hatred towards a person or entire groups that are seen to have caused them pain for no reason. This need is entirely valid- the people are, indeed, in pain when they are betrayed. However, the more betrayals, the deeper the pain – a truth that can't be seen on the outside.

Accepting our anger is the first step in being able to integrate it so that we don't inflict the same wounds on our children. When parents have not integrated their emotional trauma, they have not experienced the healing feeling of justice and fairness. As a result, they, unknowingly and unintentionally, inflict this wound on their children, as their children's behaviour will anger them extremely easily.

SHAME

Shame is a visceral reaction that is meant to stop us from repeating a certain behaviour, displaying a certain trait or owning a certain unwanted truth.

With its counterpart – "being ashamed of something", it has the highest impact on how we present ourselves in society – how we interact with other people and the "mask" we are showing others.

Its main reason is psyche fragmentation – and becoming aware of having displayed behaviour, thought patterns or emotions from one of those separated parts that have been initially pushed outside of our active awareness.

In short, psyche fragmentation is the process through which our system keeps itself safe from anything that might interfere with its proper functioning. Our psyche has the ability to split itself into parts – similar to partitions on a hard drive – and it stores the "problematic" information on these parts that are separate from our main identity. The information that is stored may contain the emotional component of specific memories, personality traits, inclinations, preferences, thoughts, thought patterns and behaviours. They may be:

- "frozen" in time – created around a deep emotional wound
- aware of the passing of time, but unaware of the main personality

- aware of the main personality, the passing of time and the current outside events

However, they are all still part of the brain, so they follow the same main rule- "ensure survival, safety, happiness". The problem is that, in designing solutions and directing behaviour, each of them takes into account only the information they have on their own "partition", completely disregarding the needs and wants of the main personality. As such, in their quest to find the best solution for survival, safety, happiness (fulfilling their own needs in accordance with their reality), they compete with the main personality over the right to make decisions. After we act out those decisions, we feel shame, as the main personality is convinced that it has done something "wrong" (usually seen as "dishonourable" – not honouring oneself).

The more fragmented our psyche, the more people, things and circumstances from our outside environment can constitute triggers for feeling the physical sensation of shame. As the natural tendency is to turn away from unpleasant triggers, shame is one of the main reasons for social isolation (it can be unconscious). Even in cases where the person seems to have a healthy social life, if the psyche is heavily fragmented, the parts that are not visible will carry with them a sense of not being seen, which leads to an ever-present and incomprehensible sense of loneliness even when surrounded by an entire social group.

Children are not born with the shame-related "feeling signature", simply because shame is the translation of thoughts, thought patterns and convictions. As such, it is closely related to the meaning attached to any situation.

Psyche fragmentation has 3 main causes:

- the process of socialisation

- high-intensity emotional wounds
- the child's chosen standards for themselves – their own decisions regarding the personality traits they choose to adopt and the ones they completely reject – their ego.

THE PROCESS OF SOCIALISATION

It is the process of teaching a child the rules of functioning in that specific family and society- the "do's" and "don'ts", to ensure successful integration within the social group.

As such, the first and foremost root cause for generalised shame is the repeated childhood experience of having been forced to hide their genuine inclinations because they did not fit into the value system of "right" and "wrong" adopted by the parents, the social group and/or the culture. Children do this automatically when they are met with painful consequences for being truthful- for saying what they like, feeling what they feel, behaving how they want to.

The process of "hiding" parts of themselves is carried out through the fragmentation of the part of the psyche that has that specific trait that led to that specific behaviour – and to push that part of the psyche into the subconscious, to ensure that it will not be "seen" anymore, so it will not be a threat to the child's belonging in that particular family and society.

The hidden traits may, actually, be, extremely beneficial for the child, and hold within them the skills needed to choose, later in life, a profession that would lead to a feeling of happiness and personal fulfilment. However, if the parents' idea of how their child should be is different from how the child really is, the child will end up having to disown and hide the parts of themselves that are different from the parents' expectations.

For example, a highly creative and artistically inclined child born in a family that values highly intellectual approaches to life will possibly have to hide the part of themselves that feels and values emotions.

As such, if any of their feelings, thoughts and/or behaviours contradict what has been taught and internalised as "right", the adult will experience the visceral reaction of **shame**. In most cases, adults are not aware of the specific "rule" they have broken, but they feel the consequences anyway.

In some cases, when children are being made to feel somehow "wrong" and "bad" by the adults around them through criticism/being reprimanded/having their ideas rejected/being sent the message that they can't do things right (e.g. a parent loses patience when the child performs a task slowly), being shamed, etc., they internalise the feeling of being "inadequate" and adopt the belief that they are "bad" or that there is something wrong with them.

Unfortunately, this belief gets triggered in social interactions, so the shame of being inadequate (wrong) seems to be ever-present, continuing in adulthood. It enhances the need to be "good", no matter what, as only through the awareness of a self that is "good" can they mitigate the persistent feeling of shame. They will not respond well to friendly observations of things that they might need to improve, as they will confuse them with "being shamed" – for them, it will mean that they're told that they have done something wrong when they shouldn't have.

HIGH-INTENSITY EMOTIONAL WOUNDS

Since the mind has decided that it is necessary to dissociate from the negative emotions and to keep them hidden, when they are visible or we make decisions from their truth, we feel the shame resulting from the conviction that we are doing something wrong, as how we felt was not ok and we shouldn't even access them, let alone display emotions, thinking patterns or behaviours resulting from them.

THE CHILD'S CHOSEN STANDARDS FOR THEMSELVES

In adulthood, we can easily identify one's chosen standards for oneself through the completion of the following statements:

I am/am not…

I never/always…

I should always/ should never…

People should always/should never…

The process of identifying with a desired trait involves a perceived threat or dislike of having the opposite one.

For example, a child growing up with a highly critical mother might decide that they don't like that trait (as it caused them pain) and that they should never be a highly critical person, to not cause the same pain in others. In consequence, whenever they display this behaviour, they feel ashamed, as they have chosen as their standard that they are not a person who criticises others.

This is the process for every chosen standard – which is not to say that it is wrong to have standards. When the person is dealing with the issue of shame, though, the opposite trait must be investigated, to uncover how having it in childhood might have been dangerous and unwanted.

As we now know, there are different reasons for fragmentation- some parts hold the knowledge of "being wrong"- opposed to the accepted value system; some parts hold the emotional wound that needed to be hidden to ensure the self-preservation of the entire system- so that it could continue experiencing life; some parts are rejected and disowned because the child decided that having them is dangerous somehow - so these parts hold within themselves a thinking pattern, behaviour or personality trait. The common thread, however, is the existence of fragmented parts within our psyche, and them being brought into our awareness by triggers gives rise to the physical sensation of shame – which is a reaction.

VI

FROM EMOTIONAL TRAUMA TO MENTAL ILLNESS. COPING MECHANISMS IN ADULTHOOD

Despite common beliefs, we never reach a state where we no longer have emotional needs.

Regardless of whether we are in childhood, teenage years, adulthood, or old age, our emotional system will continuously assess whether we are experiencing the main positive emotions connected with the fulfilment of those emotional needs- such as, but not limited to: intimacy, belonging, emotional safety, trust, etc. or whether there is a lack that needs to be addressed. The lack is indicated by emotional pain or other negative emotions like frustration, anger, envy, despair, and so on.

The emotional system is our first and main interpersonal system of communication.

The verbal, non-verbal, writing, and listening types of communication are all considered during the overall emotional translation of the received input, **but the state (feeling frequency) of our intracardiac brainwaves is the main field impacted during interpersonal communication.**

Our rational brain also plays a major role, as the IcNS decides on the corresponding emotionally translated message only after receiving and considering the thoughts and thought patterns already present in the brain. In continuation to the communication process, after receiving the input from the IcNS, the brain decides upon the most appropriate thoughts and actions to be taken in response. For example, if the emotional translation is that of feeling verbally attacked, the brain will decide upon different ways of responding depending on the meaning it has assigned to the communication and the perceived consequences – there is a different response if the brain decides that the disrespect was intended or unintended.

The beauty is that our brain has the ability to choose what it directs us to do, regardless of the emotional input received. This is very useful when there is previous emotional trauma, as the brain can make rational, helpful, and healthy decisions, whereas the emotional wounds would dictate a different, unhealthy behaviour. On the other hand, the brain may be used to completely bypass the instructions from the IcNS regarding the emotional needs required, which causes more emotional pain.

Unfortunately, this is a state of constant war between the two main systems, which does not benefit the person in the long run and leads to mental and physical health issues.

This is the state the majority of people are currently in.

As mentioned in a previous chapter, our style of relating to other people has been learned in childhood, recorded, and mapped whether it was healthy (beneficial) for us, or unhealthy (emotional wounds, unfulfilled needs, abuse). In our adult life, we unconsciously navigate towards people and situations that enable us to re-experience the exact same emotional reality, as this is what we recognise as "familiar". If our childhood environment allowed us to have a healthy emotional map of the world, we will navigate towards healthy, beneficial, and fulfilling relationships. However, if we have experienced emotional, mental, and/or physical abuse, we will re-experience in our adult relationships the same emotional wounds. Also, in adulthood we have what is called "an emotional bias" – meaning, we will automatically assign a well-known emotion (be it positive or negative) to different, diverse events.

Just a little exercise: write on a piece of paper how you felt in childhood, the role you had played in the family, how your parents interacted with you, the activities you were constantly doing and how they made you feel. Now consider how you feel in your current life and your current main relationship. Are there any similarities?

The heart brain, along with the different fragmented parts of the psyche, are continually trying to fulfil the needs they lacked in childhood, so they direct us towards similar circumstances, in order to experience the opposite and be able to fully process the open emotional wounds that are being recorded in the emotional map. From this point of view, it is all very logical. But, due to the fact that the situations and people are the same as our main attachment figures in our childhood home, there is little chance that the results are positive.

Once the emotional wounds are integrated, the adult will find themselves interested in different types of relationships, with a different relational style, that would provide a more balanced emotional life. And the most important benefit is that the brain is now free to be rational, to function how it was initially meant to function – healthy, clear of clutter, knowing that it is in charge of creating life and directing the person towards what is wanted, free to focus on the present and using more of its capacity towards analysing and finding ways for the person to thrive.

FROM EMOTIONAL TRAUMA TO MENTAL ILLNESS

As a society, we don't know yet how to deal with emotional pain. Hence, not knowing, parents will not know how to teach children about healthy ways of approaching unpleasant emotions. And this perpetuates the cycle ad infinitum.

Unpleasant emotions are an undeniable reality. Furthermore, unpleasant emotions are normal- they have a well-defined function of highlighting the awareness of an undesired experience. We should neither be afraid of, ignore, deny, reject, or fight against feeling them. As long as we allow their complete processing and/or take action towards relief, they will pass as the chemicals will fade through our bodies.

What's more important is to not miss the information they bring with them – information that sheds light on a specific aspect of our life and that will ask the brain to find ways to change the unpleasant experience.

The main 6 severe emotional traumas that lead to fragmentation are:

- Antagonism
- Betrayal

- Rejection
- Abandonment
- Humiliation
- Injustice

Since we don't know how to deal with the pain while the emotional map is being solidified, these wounds will get mapped (roughly by age 8-9) and will become part of every transmission of information from the heart to the brain until they are addressed and fully processed. Furthermore, their intensity will increase with every new experience of the same type of emotion (this is true for positive emotions, as well).

As a result, in adulthood, we often find ourselves overwhelmed by prolonged negative emotional states that we simply don't understand. Some of them are so severe that they are classified as mental and physical illnesses, even if they themselves are symptoms and consequences of emotional illnesses.

In addition, the psyche fragmentations that have at their core a severe emotional wound that has had its emotional intensity increased by trauma repetition, thus pain addition, constitute now distinct personalities whose emotional realities are being translated into thoughts once the emotional flow of information arrives from the heart. If intense enough, these partitions' "personalities" - their thoughts, feelings, and beliefs - are "leaking" into the conscious awareness, becoming the root cause for the label "mental illnesses".

For example, some of these thoughts may be experienced by the main personality as "voices", while the person does not know where they're coming from. Or, for example, other parts that have suffered grave injustice, in their need for soothing the pain, after years of suffering, might not care at all anymore about morality, values, or "what's proper", and they might display dark and violent thoughts and instructions, as they are desperate to get relief through justice.

We have to understand that their perception is REAL – as their emotional wounds are real. In this light, the individual is not necessarily mentally ill – each psyche part has reached its own conclusions, adopted its own beliefs, and has decided upon its own behaviours based on the very real emotional experience it carries within it.

As such, in the case of an individual mentally fragmented due to emotional trauma, we are not dealing with one intact psyche that is, inexplicably, having hallucinations, delusions, or irrational beliefs. We are dealing with multiple "psyche partitions" where each has its own valid reality, which has been formed following an emotionally (and mentally and/or physically) traumatising event. Just like the main brain, they follow the same instructions: survival, safety, seeking pleasure. The only problem is that, being disconnected from the main brain, there is no coherence in their collective goals, and, when the person encounters a trigger that brings into front conscious awareness a specific "partition", the indications provided will seem irrational to the main personality.

The current categorisation of mental health disorders does not take into account the fact that they all have started from emotional wounds and unfulfilled emotional needs and that the traits that differentiate them are nothing more than emotional trauma consequences and their coping mechanisms. In other words, we categorise them as per their chosen modality of reacting to their pain, instead of categorising them as per their emotional root cause/trauma (it may

be simple or complex) and sub-categorising them as per their chosen coping mechanisms.

From an outsider's perspective- the problem with misunderstanding them in other people is the fact that we consider them "mental illnesses" from the beginning and judge them from the premise that the only valid reality is our own, so they should perceive and react to the same consensus reality as us.

In consequence, we address them as if they were, indeed, inexplicable dysfunctionalities of the same complete psyche that shares the same reality with us. We have to take into account that the thoughts, language, and behaviours they display are in direct correlation with the emotions they receive from the IcNS, which they translate and react to. Those emotions convey a reality that we cannot perceive, which does not make it any less real for the individual experiencing them.

Sometimes, they completely take over the main personality, so it looks as if the entire psyche is dysfunctional. However, if we get access to their core trauma, we easily notice that they are independent parts that may live in an everlasting present, may have the same emotional and mental age as when they were first traumatised, and may not even have had their cognition processes completed yet.

As a result of our lack of knowledge of how to integrate these parts in the main psyche when they first disconnected, the majority of people have several separate "partitions". This can be easily observed when we have contradictory desires. The further disconnected these parts' emotional reality from the main personality's perception of reality, the more the tendency to be labelled as "mental illness".

However, the brain has the ability to access at will any of these "psyche partitions", to listen to them, to identify their pain, and to take the necessary actions to diminish it. By integrating the emotional wounds, bringing them back into the consensus reality, and, when needed, adapting one's own behaviours to fulfil their emotional needs, we change the emotional information recorded in the IcNS, which will change how the brain translates it and reacts to it.

EMOTIONAL WOUNDS AND THEIR COPING MECHANISMS IN ADULTHOOD

In order to diminish the toxic impact of these persistent painful emotional states on the proper functioning of the entire system, the system itself employs a series of coping mechanisms. Below is a very short list of such mechanisms (the reasons are not limited to the ones mentioned):

- internally-devised
  - mental
    - psyche fragmentation – it can have any number of behaviours, from keeping the pain in the subconscious to forget about it to attacking the main personality to ensure the adoption of the "right" behaviour
    - mental patterns - the beliefs considered to be "irrational", but that are designed to keep the person safe from re-experiencing the pain
    - repressed memories – memories preserved inside the separated parts, to keep the system safe from their awareness and the consequential pain

- positive focus - that takes attention away from the pain
- mental confusion/fog – to derail oneself from the awareness of the pain of emotional neglect/ lack of physical touch or severe physical abuse
- suicide ideation – to provide momentary relief from despair/anger/powerlessness

- behaviours
    - physical movement – to flood the system with endorphins, to ease the pain, without addressing the pain
    - sex – to create momentary pain relief through the release of endorphins and/or the illusion of having human connection
    - ADHD – to diminish anxiety overflow
    - Cutting – to diminish the pain, to cleanse, to ask for help when the emotions are not seen;
    - Murdering – to feel momentary relief from intense anger, humiliation, injustice through fulfilling the need for justice and personal power
    - Raping – to regain a momentary sense of control and personal power
    - Psychopathy – voluntarily stopping the main system of interpersonal communication to keep oneself safe from re-experiencing feelings of betrayal/injustice/humiliation. Illusions of grandeur to counteract the trauma of being made to feel extremely unimportant by main attachment figures
    - Over-eating
    - Over-fasting

- somatic responses
  - auto-immune disorders
  - cancer
  - other physical illnesses

- externally-provided coping mechanisms:
  - relationship styles
    - Narcissism – to ensure survival by fighting for your needs - learned in a family where no one seemed to care if your emotional needs were met;
    - Co-dependency – to ensure survival by manipulating others to have your needs met – learned in a family where no one seemed to care if your emotional needs were met
  - chemical substances – opioids, alcohol, stimulants, sedatives, etc. – to numb or overflow feelings like utter loneliness, powerlessness, disappointment, despair, and so on;
  - information (to by-pass)
    - religion – used for a certain enlightened meaning to the pain, to help counteract it through perceived usefulness and the positive feeling of knowing oneself to be "good"
    - spirituality – used to diminish the importance of pain to diminish the perceived intensity

○ psychology- using the labels on the pain to provide a positive feeling of control that creates the impression of safety

It is necessary to mention that some of the above – like positive focus, spirituality, body movement, psychology, religion – are very useful in their healthy expression.

A different way of organising them would be the following:

- diminishing – that diminish pain awareness
- over-compensating – that flood the system with positive emotion
- stopping – that attempt to interrupt the heart-brain flow of information (some anti-depression medication that numbs the emotional perception).

Nonetheless, they are all coping mechanisms – that will no longer be employed once the emotional reality they are trying to cover is fully acknowledged, processed, and improved.

Regarding the somatic responses, some of them are categorised as physical illnesses, which does not negate their role in helping the physical body cope with pain.

THE RELATIONSHIP IcNS-CNS-PHYSICAL ILLNESS

There are multiple possibilities of how the physical body can become sick in response to an emotional or mental root cause.

1. As long as the IcNS has unprocessed traumatic emotional information, it will continuously transmit it to the brain and the Autonomic Nervous System. In turn, corresponding thoughts and corresponding chemicals will be created and sent into the body – to the corresponding areas that are recorded as the specific areas where that type of emotion is to be felt (this information is encoded in the IcNS from birth, as presented in a previous chapter). In time, the accumulation becomes toxic, and the physical body starts showing symptoms in the form of physical illnesses. Once the information stored in the IcNS is changed (by fulfilling the emotional need that provides the opposite positive emotion necessary for that experience to lower its intensity sufficiently so as to be safely archived), the body will no longer be flooded with those chemicals.

2. Situations where the experience was so traumatising that the emotion is basically blocked in the body, mid-circulation, stopping the correct functioning of sensors present in that area. In addition to allowing the emotion to fully circulate (emotional integration), somatic therapy - such as massage or acupuncture - is a very good therapeutic method to speed up the process.

3. Recurrent negative beliefs that get transmitted to the heart brain and get translated into emotions will, in time, affect

the physical area where those emotions are felt – through the mechanism indicated

It seems that the heart has the ability to translate feeling brainwaves into emotions – which means that it has the ability to translate energy fields into emotions. We are currently waiting for further scientific research regarding the intracardiac brainwaves, their energy fields, and their impact on the physical body, as they might have a significant role to play in physical illnesses.

What is currently presented is that the emotion of love vibrates at the 500Hz frequency, while that of fear vibrates at 100hz, anger at 150hz, and shame at 20hz.

CANCER

It is the coping mechanism of a part of the psyche (with the associated body part that it governs) that is in such deep pain that it feels it will die if it does not separate itself from the central command system. The perception is that its needs are completely overlooked and that it is left alone to die- so, in order to survive, it decides to take control of its own "life".

The outside situation consists of a person who refuses to change a specific painful reality that has been experienced for a long time – be it a negative family environment, un-fulfilling work choices, past unprocessed trauma (unrecog-nised, denied), a feeling of lack of love or appreciation, etc.

After it separates, like any other new-born life, it will revert the physical cells of the body region where the pain is supposed to be experienced as per the IcNS rules of functioning (as it was previously presented, the IcNS ensures that the same emotions are experienced by all people in the same specific body regions) to their undifferentiated state (before they specialised to be part of a specific organ) and will start to grow- fulfilling the first instinct of any living organism. Thus, treatment involves accessing that part's reality, listening to its pain, needs, and requests, and convincing it of our love for it- showing it that we care enough as to change the emotional reality it kept experiencing. The "convincing" part must be accompanied by clear, decisive, and sustained action – as we are already dealing with a separate living organism that felt deeply betrayed by the central being that was supposed to care for it – so it does not trust the person anymore. **The painful emotional reality MUST be improved and MUST be sustained over time** – otherwise, the person will have an internal "war" between a main system that wants to maintain control by annihilating the chaotic "part" and a separate "part" that has "rebelled" as it had nothing left to lose.

If we want to survive cancer, we have to stop killing parts of ourselves and, instead, show compassion to the entirety of our being.

VII

EMOTIONAL TRAUMA
IN CHILDREN

The most crucial part of raising a child is tending to their emotional well-being.

There is this misconception that children forget, so there is no consequence for dismissive or aggressive behaviour and speech towards them. Although this widely adopted belief saves some parents and other adults from guilt and responsibility for their own actions and behaviours, it is actually entirely inaccurate.

Children may not remember from one day to another- or even from one moment to another- what was talked about or what happened, but they have recorded how the event felt, along with the rest of the external output and the age-informed thoughts that their brain created as a translation of that emotional reality.

As such, this emotional information is added up to the rest of their recorded life experience, creating the blueprint for their emotional reality and emotional "palette" available for them for the rest of their lives, along with the beliefs and thought patterns created after this blueprint.

Relative to the subject of emotional trauma, we must highlight the most common misconceptions, which, even if are not spelt out, are part of the hidden belief systems that drive some adults' behaviour towards children in our current society:

Children are not pets, are not dolls, are not "clay" to mould, and neither are they stupid. They are not their parents' property, nor are they "in the process of becoming people".

Children ARE people from the moment they are born and, thus, they have the right to be seen and treated with the same respect and emotional consideration shown towards human beings that have reached adulthood.

Of course, keeping in mind that the most important aspect to be shown consideration towards is **their emotional reality.**

In a society that praises only the intellect, it is easy to dismiss, overlook, overpower, control, disapprove of, belittle, despise, punish, laugh at or plainly not believe the feelings and words of those who are in the process of creating that intellect.

If we want to be able to reach states of joy, happiness, fulfilment, later in life, as a society, we must start valuing the blueprint for our thinking patterns, beliefs and future coping behaviours. As children, we record everything our parents, siblings, other relatives, friends make us feel and based on that, we create our thinking processes and beliefs, and we adopt our future behaviours.

We only need coping behaviours for feelings and emotions that we think we cannot change- because we learned that we couldn't.

As such, what you will most easily observe in children (but it is valid for adults, too), is that they will try to make you feel exactly how you make them feel.

So, if you don't like how they're acting, but you know that their behaviour is in response to yours, you have the option to purposefully change your behaviour to elicit a different emotion in them, which will then drive a different behaviour from their part.

If you want respect, you have to find ways to make them feel respected.

If you want love, take actions that they translate as love coming from you.

When you want consistency, you have to show consistency.

If you want them to do what you want when you want it- they will retaliate and **make you feel how they feel** when you try to force them to do something they don't want to do when they don't want to do it. Usually, that is a feeling of angry powerlessness- they will try and make you feel like there's nothing you can do to remediate the situation.

It is not desirable, but it is what it is.

When you don't allow them to choose what to do, they will become inflexible and make you feel how it feels to deal with an inflexible person. That is- because they do not have yet the concept of "painful or dangerous consequences", so they do not understand you- nor the reason for your requests. Now there is a perfect opportunity for you, yourself, to question your own reasons: are you trying to keep your child safe from experiencing pain or are you trying to make your own life easier, disregarding their own need for learning?

Because the best time for children to grasp the concept that actions have consequences is when those consequences are relatively minor.

For example, what is the consequence for them if they run out in the snow with no coat on? They will feel the cold in a few minutes, and they will learn that they do not like it – that is part of the learning process. Next time, they'll remember.

It's much better than being 13 and not having the habit of thinking about the consequences of their actions.

Up until age 8-9, children function mainly from their primary system, with the rational system gradually interfering between stimuli and reaction. Their behaviour makes total sense – they are following their internal emotional compass towards what feels good, without fully understanding the notion of "negative feeling". Fear is something WE LEARN.

Attempts at controlling a child's behaviour is a much more serious offensive action, as it has devastating effects on that child's entire future life.

Shame, guilt, punishments of all sorts, emotional withdrawals or bursts of negative emotions and physical abuse towards them – anger, rage, yelling, blaming- are all current attempts at controlling a child's behaviour -and they are all very damaging and abusive. They create the blueprint for adults that perpetuate that pain onto others in society. By abusing our children, we create in them the emotions that they will later have towards us. **Parents seldom consider that their children have the right to get angry for being made to feel negative emotions, like an adult would.** They punish that anger, too. However, children DO GROW UP eventually and they REMEMBER how they were treated.

Emotional neglect is abuse, too- so, the method of raising children without caring at all about their behaviour is actually creating the wound of being abandoned- at which point, children will do anything to attract attention- even mistreat other people just to get a reaction from their parents.

Now, it is entirely understandable that it is almost impossible in this society- due to how it is currently structured and the limited knowledge about the emotional wounds we ourselves carry from our own childhood- to entirely refrain from reacting when your child triggers you. But it is not that child's fault.

On one hand, the current societal structure places parents in the impossible position of caring for their children on their own, alone, while also ensuring the continuation of the rest of their lives. That is not only unfair, but also extremely cruel, as parents are over-whelmed, emotionally drained, and, on top of that, lose financial support as they cannot provide their services for society – **as if raising a child is not done FOR the continuation of that said community and society at large.**

On the other hand, the fact that a child's normal behaviour is a consistent trigger for a parent's previous emotional wounds- does not mean that the child does something wrong and that, consequen-tially, they should change. Every parent on this planet complains about the same behaviour from children- does that mean that we, as a species, are all born "wrong", and we should be made to change into something acceptable – or that we haven't yet understood the normal processes that drive our behaviours in childhood?

It is the parents' responsibility to heal their own emo-tional wounds, so that they may be able to get out of the reactive state and connect with the child's reality- to under-stand the unwanted behaviour and provide guidance with care and compassion.

Parents who feel strong and prolonged negative emotions in reaction to something their child does or needs are usually over-whelmed – at which point, they should really strive to find additional help – and lots of additional help is needed in raising a child anyway! If the negative emotions persist, they should avail of the emotional trauma therapy, in order to diminish their intensity and ensure that their emotional reaction and ensuing behaviours are appropriate. Taking the easy way out - taking advantage of their superior position - will only ensure the escalation of that conflict, be it overt or be it transferred towards a more passive-aggressive approach. And we have sufficient conflict anyway.

When a parent comes into therapy and works towards paying attention to and integrating their own childhood emotional wounds, they realise that the relationship with their children greatly improves at the same time.

HOW DO CHILDREN COPE WITH AN EMOTIONALLY DIFFICULT REALITY?

We often see children who are happy, playing around, smiling, and we conclude that they must be emotionally healthy, as well. However, what we observe in specific moments is not representative of their entire life experience. Since the main activity in childhood is emotional learning, children accumulate experiences, record how they feel in the body, assign meaning to each of the emotions, and then move on to the next experience. This means that they may have recorded experiences with very unpleasant sensory and emotional components, and they can still laugh and smile and play, as their reality is felt moment by moment.

The older they get, though, the more there is a cohesion between all their emotional memories, creating what we, as adults, experience as a baseline emotional state- the overall feeling result of the negative and positive feeling intensity of all of our life experiences (whether we consciously remember them or not). The more emotionally difficult experiences we have recorded in our IcNS, the more emotionally heavier our adult life is.

There is a straightforward connection between parents' emotional states and their children's emotional and mental reality. Parents with suppressed or expressed high-intensity negative emotions will create those emotions in their children, which they will then display through different behaviours. For example, parents with unaddressed anxiety may have children with ADHD. Or, parents with repressed anger may have children who display violent bursts of anger. The explanation is that the child feels overwhelmed and tries to cope as best as they can- by regulating their anxiety/anger through sensory integration and tension release. When the level of anxiety/anger is lowered in their family environments, the child's nervous system starts to calm down, getting out of that state of extreme stress and into a more peaceful experience. Bringing the child into therapy without first addressing and improving the emotional reality in their environment, i.e. without treating their parents' emotional wounds and relationship style, brings little improvement to the child's mental state, as any dysregulation, even treated with the emotional integration therapy, gets re-activated by interacting with the parents in the unhealthy environment.

This is a reality for the rest of the emotions, too.

Of course, this is a wonderful thing when the prevalent emotional reality in the family is healthy.

Some of the most traumatising childhood experiences are the following:

- emotional neglect – when the child's emotional life is completely overlooked as if it does not exist and it is of no importance. As such, there is very little emotional connection in the family environment, even if all the other aspects of upbringing are provided. The basic emotional needs that can be fulfilled only through other people (like intimacy and closeness) are completely overlooked, so the adult does not even know that something was missing in their childhood. However, their baseline emotional state is painful, without the possibility of pinpointing a real cause.
- physical neglect – occurs when small children are not embraced, are not held or caressed. Moving from always being in physical contact (in the womb) to never being touched is registered in the heart brain as a diminishing of a good-feeling emotion. Its translation in the CNS resembles a command to "shrink" the brain- resulting in physical pain and mental confusion/fog.
- emotional invalidation – when the child's emotions are downplayed, ignored or dismissed. They can see that their emotion bothers the parent, so they will convince themselves that having that emotion is not ok. In adulthood, they will automatically go against their own emotions, which will cause them to actually increase in intensity.
- gaslighting – when the child is being told that what they feel, see or hear and the meaning they assign to it is not an accurate depiction of what is happening, that they are completely wrong, and that reality is different. This is the case where a child is being hurt by a parent's behaviour or words, but they are told that the parent loves them. The emotional translation of the parent's behaviour towards them does not match the emotion the parent asks the child to have. In adulthood, when they are contradicted, these people will become

confused and will doubt their own perceptions, memory and even their sanity. They will often ask others for their opinion regarding specific events in order to decide what the truth is and how they should feel or act in relation to it or they will become the exact opposite, avid seekers of truth in everything they, others or society at large thinks, says or does.

The most important realisation is that all childhood emotional and mental issues are the direct result of the emotional translation of their external environment and the meaning attached to it.

In therapy, after integrating the child's emotional trauma, which will cause the improvement of their mental issues, it must be identified if the external cause for that emotional wound is still present in the child's environment. Failure to remove or improve the external experience will result in a continuous re-traumatisation and the wound will be, again, recorded as a valid experience to be kept in the child's emotional map of the world and used in the blueprint of their mental map, which will later be the reason for adopting specific coping mechanisms – resulting in mental and physical issues in their adult life.

The logical conclusion is that a child with emotional, mental and/or behavioural issues is a definite symptom of a dysfunctional family environment, thus, the entire family is in need of attention. The parents are responsible for the child's **entire** well-being, and they can provide a healthy life only by ensuring that they, themselves, are emotionally healthy.

PSYCHOPATHY

It is a coping mechanism for complex trauma where the child feels like the caregiver **does not love them at all** – and the child chooses to cut off the heart-brain connection - to keep themselves safe from feeling the incredibly painful emotional reality of not being loved – observed at a time when all they know, feeling-wise, is the feeling of intense connection (the feeling of love that was mapped in the womb) to their main attachment figures. Hence, they will display shallow emotions later in life. Additionally, in doing so, the child also shuts off **the main inter-human communication system that would lead to feeling empathy and a sense of connection with other people.** Without it, the person identified as having "psychopathic tendencies" will no longer feel a sense of species similarity and belonging- it will lead to a sense of complete separateness - so they will act as a predator, similar to how humans have acted towards other animal species.

From the behaviours displayed in adulthood, we must conclude that they have experienced antagonistic, injustice or humiliation trauma in their early childhood, as these lead to aggressive tendencies on top of the feeling of not being loved. They also have symptoms of betrayal trauma- when the abuser is expected to love the child, but they harm them instead.

The reason that anger gets through the blockage is because anger is perceived as a more powerful state than the trauma experienced – it improves the overall emotional reality.

Lack of guilt or remorse indicates generalised extreme hate (which is a cover emotion for extreme pain) – which is congruent with bystander trauma resulting from extrapolating the caregiver's role in the abuse to the entire species.

An individual may have one psychopathic part (kept hidden) and several other parts that help them adapt to society, as the purpose is to survive and thrive. That is the modality they found to be able to blend in so easily, and that is why it is so difficult to identify individuals with psychopathic traits when observing their behaviour in society at large, excluding the reality of family dynamics.

In society, instead of "hiding" some of their vulnerable parts, these individuals have decided to make use of them, as they learned that they can manipulate people through the artificial display of certain emotions and behaviours. As such, they will employ behaviours that get "translated" by other people through emotions that will "draw them in" and use this sense of deep friendship or respect as a "safety net", should their psychopathic part ever be in danger of being seen.

These individuals may have, actually, an extremely high emotional potential, with a deep innate sense of family/ tribe/community, which might be the reason they experienced betrayal pain with such a high intensity.

TEENAGE SUICIDE

The mental constructs of an adult who chooses to commit suicide are the result of the feeling of despair, a total loss of hope of having the power to change something in their internal or external world. We must, however, highlight, that this feeling might be the reality of only some of the internal parts created in the psyche following traumatising events, parts that are kept separate, with their emotional and mental realities frozen in that starting point, continuously in pain, unable to see or feel the reality experienced by the rest of the psyche. As a result, those parts conclude that the only way to diminish the pain – and the only power they have- is to just let go of it altogether. Death is seen as RELIEF and deliverance from despair.

In some cases, following serious emotional neglect trauma in childhood, adults have as their baseline emotional reality a feeling of utter despair/pain/loss of hope/lack of joy/lack of meaning in life, which they cannot understand and from which they cannot run. In this case, too, suicide is seen as RELIEF and giving up a battle where the real enemy is unknown. Unfortunately, the parents have no idea how to help, even if they desperately want to, as they, in their turn, are not aware of what they did not provide to the child who is now an adult.

Suicide ideation provides a momentary relief of emotional peace. It is, sometimes, an attempt at solving the emotional burden of injustice trauma (when death is perceived as a punishment for the ones that caused the deep hurt, but any attempt at hurting them back emotionally in real life seems to have no effect, as they prove to be completely emotionally unavailable and in their own "bubble reality". In consequence, the only way to have justice is by hurting them back through extreme loss).

Since the root cause for the feeling of despair and powerlessness is not visible to the people on the outside, the suicidal person is, in most cases, not understood and completely invalidated in their view of the world. However, their experience is entirely real- it's just that it's kept on a separate "brain partition", along with the initial memories and all the additional painful life events that are added up onto the first trauma, deepening the emotional wound and serving as confirmation of the attached meaning. When these memories are triggered by outside sensory perceptions (a word, an event, a person, a situation, etc.), the parts in despair take over the emotional system and the psyche, and their mental constructs begin to be present in that person's mind. **The issue is that, by virtue of being kept separate from the main personality, they have needs that the person themselves, along with the other people around them, don't understand and can't fulfil, on top of people being unable to connect with those parts, thus enhancing the deep feeling of being utterly alone and misunderstood.**

Emotional Integration therapy enables us to reach out to those parts and heal their emotional wounds, thus making their reality a lot less painful, bringing in hope and personal power.

When it comes to teenagers, the process is exactly the same. The usual reasons are:

- being continuously attacked by an aggressive parent, with no possibility to leave the environment;
- having been emotionally, mentally or physically abused, their reality is completely denied by the parents and siblings, the teenager being continuously gaslit;
- being pushed into the position of "the family's scapegoat", thus being used as a let-out for their entire family's dysfunctions (all the blame for different family issues is put on them);
- having been sexually abused, there is deep shame and desire to stop the intrusive thoughts and feelings. Shock, injustice, being undefended and alone, the world is utterly unsafe and there is a deep desire to not be part of it anymore;
- Being continuously emotionally attacked either by direct verbal abuse or through attacking their standing and reputation (either by a parent or a group of friends/colleagues, etc) there

is the desire to have revenge on the attacker while getting out of a situation perceived as deeply shameful.

There are many other variations of the above situations, however, the ever-present reason is always found in an outside experience, be it in the teenage years or having started in childhood and being heightened later on.

In any case of teenage suicide, our justice department should identify the perpetrators - to send them towards mandatory therapy to reduce their aggressive tendencies and prevent them from subjecting, even unknowingly, other innocent people to the same abusive behaviours.

A CHILD'S PERCEPTION OF SOCIETY

As adults, when we are going through "tough times", we turn to our friends and family for support.

As children are just starting their life journey, they feel they belong in the society where they are born. By seeing themselves as part of the group of people surrounding them (not only family but ALL the people they know and all the adults that see them, that live in the same building block, neighbourhood, city, etc.), they expect the group to see them and help them when needed. Every time a child is attacked, abused, in visible pain, and the adults around them DO NOT HELP, the child experiences "betrayal trauma", which is another name for "bystander trauma". (For example, when a parent is verbally or physically abusing their child and the parent's adult friend does not say anything in the child's defence). This human expectation that the society one belongs into is bound by the moral laws to provide help, assistance, protection to children derives from our history as primates being part of a group and, later, a tribe. It is deeply encoded in our DNA. So, when adults DON'T PROTECT children, they are basically going against their own human nature.

When these children with betrayal trauma grow up, the deep pain has been covered by the emotion of hate, in many cases directed towards entire groups, with no regard to individuals, who are not seen as separate but hated altogether.

HOW TO RAISE EMOTIONALLY HEALTHY CHILDREN?

First of all, parents must remember that children experience life through their emotions- these are completely real. In any interaction, consider how the child feels- and strive to make the experience a positive one. Also, smile more at your child- it will make them feel loved, accepted, good, a bringer of happiness.

In infancy, crying indicates that the child wants something- and "wanting" is the same as "needing" at that very fragile age. It is extremely damaging for a child's emotional system to be ignored when crying – as the repeated experience is mapped in the IcNS as a "missing connection" – which is the first step towards psychopathy.

When a negative feeling is identified, consider it as valid and important, as it is a piece of information for the child. Ask questions- "how do you feel?", "why?", "what made you feel this way?", and validate the child's emotions, as you would feel the same way in their situation. Also, bear in mind that the child is just starting to learn about their emotions- how they feel, their names, what they mean, etc. Help the child identify the feeling, validate it, find what they don't like and what they would like instead and, most importantly, **assist them in finding a way to solve the situation** that is causing them that emotional distress. This will not only provide emotional relief but will teach the child that they have control over their emotional reality

Say "sorry", show kindness, and, most importantly, listen to what the child has to tell you. It is most likely that the negative feeling is informing the child that they do not like something- and that the particular experience must be changed. This is the basis for the child's ability to choose good-feeling experiences later in life. If the parents override this information and don't allow the possibility of choice, they are just condemning the child to a limited and painful adult life.

It must be highlighted, though, that the modality of raising children must be drastically reviewed and improved. Parents need more resources, proper directions and new societal arrangements that allow them to preserve their emotional well-being while ensuring that their children are still being loved and taken care of.

With the current social structure of most family environments comprised only of two adults and, occasionally, one or two grandparents, the parents get overwhelmed, and the child grows up, more or less, in emotional scarcity, which leads to a very limited emotional palette – and many wounds. In contrast to the large groups of children playing together, now we see individual parents accompanying their small children outside to play- alone.

Since our children are our future, ensuring the mapping of the healthiest and most complete emotional system is the base for the healthiest progress of our race. This leads to the necessity of adapting our societal structure to allow for and encourage the creation of small social groups – micro-communities- that would provide parents and children with the much-needed emotional and physical support.

VIII

ADDITIONAL
POSITIVE
CONSEQUENCES OF
EMOTIONAL TRAUMA
INTEGRATION

WHAT IS YOUR REAL AGE?

We often hear people complain that they feel older than they are- and we can actually see it on their physical body – they do, indeed, seem somehow "older".

One of the unexpected consequences of emotional trauma integration is its impact on the concept of AGE.

It has been noticed that the perception of age is not related to time but to the emotional perception of one's own reality and life.

In other words, the more positive a person's baseline is, the younger they feel – and the more negative/painful the baseline, the older they feel.

This is logical, in a way- since the feeling of "youthfulness" is translated by the emotions we experienced in childhood: happiness, curiosity, hope, excitement, boldness, and so on.

The baseline is the sum of the state of one's emotional map and the current perception of their day-to-day life.

The less painful the information kept in the heart brain, the younger the heart brain feels.

Feelings are the for IcNS the equivalent of brain waves for the brain- while emotions seem to be the equivalent of thoughts. So, the overall heart brainwave state is obviously influenced by both the information recorded and the current feeling wave.

As such, to speed up the process of getting to feel younger, one has to address the painful information recorded – yes- but it is also necessary to focus positively on the present (and preferably project positive thoughts regarding the future).

Carrying less emotional baggage and creating good feeling states every day is what ensures the feeling of being young, regardless of the age counted in years.

IcNS IN MEN VS. WOMEN

If we take into account the information from the recently published IcNS imaging, we can conclude that there are differences in emotional perception based on gender – in other words, men and women may translate the same outside experience with emotions of different intensities. Also, considering the difference in hormone levels and hormonal cycle (24 hours for men and 28 days for women), we notice that it provides support for the yin-yang concept from Traditional Chinese Medicine.

Additionally, since the hormonal cycle- which is a type of circulation- is shorter in men than in women, it might indicate that the emotional circulation mirrors a difference in length.

Hence, we may consider that William Golding was indeed right when he said: "Whatever you give a woman, she will make greater. If you give her sperm, she'll give you a baby. If you give her a house, she'll give you a home. If you give her groceries, she'll give you a meal. If you give her a smile, she'll give you her heart. She multiplies and enlarges what is given to her."

From the above analysis, we can draw the following conclusion: when a man initiates an outside experience, he will process the emotional translation much faster- according to his circulation pattern. A woman will receive the outside stimuli, translate them into emotions, and then, because her arrangement of intracardiac neurons and the emotional circulation length are different (supported by her hormonal levels), she will feel a higher intensity for a longer period of time. The emotions will be translated into thoughts and consequential behaviours, which will, then, be shown as a reaction – "answering" to the man's action - completing, thus, the inter-personal communication.

These seem to be two quite different types of emotional energies – one that initiates, and the other one that amplifies and sends the amplified feelings back to the initiator.

Women are perfectly designed to be able to enhance and hold the emotion of unconditional love so that the child in the uterus gets the IcNS mapped with the first and most important feeling signature/emotion - love- that fulfils the need for connection, while men are perfectly designed to take swift action based on their emotional information - action that moves them forward to the next experience.

Anatomically, it seems that the female body is better suited to support the processes of the heart brain, while the male one is better suited to fulfil the processes of the CNS. Depending on our intention and focus, we can choose which brain's "specialty" we need and use at a specific time.

The above theory might, at first glance, seem to suggest that women's role is insignificant. However, please remember every-thing you have read until now- and notice the huge role the heart brain has in the overall quality of our lives- and the massive impact a wounded heart has on the brain's ability to be rational.

The same as the heart and the brain, men and women are meant to work together, harmoniously, for the greater accomplishment of a life well lived and a healthy human population.

IX

IMPLICATIONS FOR SOCIETY AT LARGE

PSYCHOLOGY

The most important takeaway from this book is the fact that we, as a species, have an emotional system managed by a separate brain that works in tandem with our main brain when making decisions. We can consider that we have different managing centres for the affective and the logical functions of the human nervous system: an "affective" brain and a "rational" or "logical" brain.

If our emotional system is faulty – our logical reasoning will be, too- and they will both lead to a painful existence.

In some cases, due to intense wounds, our psyche will create separate partitions and then, the person, when reaching adulthood, will make decisions from these separate wounded psyche partitions (now, full distinct personalities).

On an individual level, these wounded parts- **that still have the emotional age of a child** – will make decisions that will lead to perpetuating the pain and unintentionally hurting other members of society – including their children- while fully believing that they are keeping the person safe from pain.

Unfortunately, as things stand now, with emotions seen as "lower" than logic and the placement of physical needs first, we are dealing with an unprecedented wave of moral perversion in our society, a direct result of unrecognised and untreated emotional wounds. The state of war between emotions and rationality is completely illogical, since they are both vital human systems, and advice to have your mind win over your emotions is a coping mechanism for this lack of recognition of the existence of emotional wounds carried with us from childhood, that lead to seemingly "irrational" behaviours. Treat the wounds and the mental and behavioural patterns will become healthier.

However, we must highlight the vital role the mind plays in our life progression. The mind, with its physical counterpart – the brain- is responsible for creating the thoughts and taking the actions that will create MORE life. **There wouldn't be any progress if the mind would not be respected and allowed to fulfil its role in its entirety and with authority.**

POLITICS/LEADERSHIP

On a societal level, these wounded parts - **that still have the emotional age of a child** – will prompt the rise of leaders who seek power from a place of trauma. When threatened, they will be incapable of showing empathy, as the fear of re-experiencing the initial trauma of powerlessness will override the main personality. On a group level, this materialises in the ability to wage war against entire groups of people, without empathy for the general suffering – neither of their compatriots nor their "enemies".

When similar wounds are present at a societal level, that society is extremely easy to be manipulated by artificially deepening the initial wounds to make the system kick into the cover emotions-HATE, ANGER, APATHY – and then use the entire group/society against the chosen target. We can easily find examples in our current global events, where citizens' fears are being used and heightened by the media, with the result that entire groups fight among themselves without a clear image of the expected results. That is due to the truth that the conflict isn't, actually, their initial trauma.

SOCIETAL HEALTH

If we want to start raising healthy children, we have to turn to our highly empathic part of the population. When empaths heal the emotional wounds that had made them empaths in the first place, they still keep their ability – and so, they will be able to fully attune to their children's emotional needs.

Emotionally healed empaths are the parents we need in order to raise the first generation of emotionally healthy humans.

JUSTICE SYSTEM

Since the purpose of incarceration is to ensure that the offenders regret their actions and will not repeat them anymore (on top of assisting the victims with treating their injustice trauma caused by the offender's actions), their willingness to participate in emotional integration therapy during their sentence is the best proof that the purpose of the "punishment" is completely fulfilled. Where the offenders are unwilling to become less of a threat to society, it is a statement that they have no interest in not causing harm anymore, which disqualifies them from being released into society until such time as they choose to become a safe element.

INDIVIDUAL EMPOWERMENT

We have to remember that, when an action is taken from a triggered pain, resolving the current issue will not make the pain disappear. The next trigger will cause the same pain, until the initial wound is integrated. Then, the same event will no longer be a trigger for pain.

This is how one achieves personal power and takes rational charge of their life.

Our central nervous system is extremely important, as it has the ability to make us feel whatever emotions we want – through the conscious and intentional creation of thoughts. In consequence, what we pay attention to and what we allow to dictate and create thoughts in our minds is what we allow to dictate the quality of our lives.

In conclusion, if you are looking to be in charge of your own life – the following are some of the points to pay attention to:

- Have a healthy emotional map – so, integrate your emotional wounds
- Focus on the present, do the emotional work when triggered
- Focus on the positive – to create positive emotions in your life
- Notice the negative – these events/emotions are indicators for wounds in your heart brain that need to be processed. The

more you ignore them, the more they'll negatively impact
your life

- Use your mind to imagine a positive future – it creates the
emotion of hope
- Use your logical brain to analyse, create, plan, execute – it
gives a sense of safety and control over your own life
- Breathe- deeply
- Pay close attention to your body – where it hurts, there's a
wound- treat it
- Use your senses to create pleasant experiences – as they get
translated by the heart brain into positive emotions (through
music, colours, touch, movement, etc.)
- Use the inter-human communication system to have access
to the positive emotions that arise only through relationships

And, most of all – remember that there is no need to cope with
pain anymore. We are all here to enjoy life.

BIBLIOGRAPHY

1. Armour, J. A., & Ardell, J. L. (2004). *Neurocardiology: anatomical and functional principles.* Complementary and Alternative Medicine, 4, 14.
2. Armour, J.A. *Intrinsic Cardiac Neurons*, Journal of Cardiovascular Electrophysiology, Canada, 1991 **https://doi.org/10.1111/j.1540-8167.1991.tb01330.x**
3. Cannon, W.B. *Bodily Changes in Pain, Hunger, Fear and Rage: An Account of Recent Researches into the Function of Emotional Excitement*; D. Appleton & Company: New York, NY, USA, 1915; p. 92. [**Google Scholar**]
4. Winnicott, D. W. *Mirror-role of Mother and Family in Child Development.* The Collected Works of D. W. Winnicott: Volume 8, 1967 – 1968, oct 2016 https://academic.oup.com/book/1195/chapter-abstract/140034320?redirectedFrom=fulltext
5. Epel, E. S., McEwen, B., Seeman, T., Matthews, K., Castellazzo, G., Brownell, K. D., ... & Ickovics, J. R. (2000). *Stress and body shape: stress-induced cortisol secretion is consistently greater among women with central fat.* Psychosomatic medicine, 62(5), 623-632.
6. Garfinkel, S. N., Zorab, E., Navon, I., Yeshurun, Y., & Dupont, S. (2017). *Body-mind communication in the somatic nervous system.* Frontiers in Human Neuroscience, 11, 126. doi: 10.3389/fnhum.2017.00126

http://www.alternativemedicinenis.com.au/Organ%20Transplants%20and%20Cellular%20Memories.pdf

https://www.sciencealert.com/scientists-discover-a-new-type-of-cell-in-the-heart-that-regulates-its-rhythm

7. Kikel-Coury NL, Brandt JP, Correia IA, O'Dea MR, DeSantis DF, Sterling F, et al. (2021) *Identification of astroglia-like cardiac nexus glia that are critical regulators of cardiac development and function.* PLoS Biol 19(11): e3001444. **https://doi.org/10.1371/journal.pbio.3001444**

8. Langley, J.N. *The Autonomic Nervous System Part I;* W Heffer and Sons Ltd.: Cambridge, UK, 1921; p. 80.

9. LeDoux, J. E. (1996). *The emotional brain: The mysterious underpinnings of emotional life.* Simon and Schuster.

10. Medow, H. (2016). *Neuroplasticity. Biology of psychotherapy.* CreateSpace Independent Publishing Platform, 2016

11. Nield, D. *A new kind of cell discovered in the heart seems to be critical for your heartbeat* Extracted from ScienceAlert Journal, 22 November 2021

12. Nummenmaa, L., Glerean E., Hari R., Hietanen J. (2013) *Bodily maps of emotions.* Psychological and cognitive sciences, 111 (2) 646-651
https://doi.org/10.1073/pnas.1321664111

13. O'Leary, K., Bylsma, L. M., Rottenberg, J., & Jarrett, R. B. (2009). *Parents' depression history and children's diagnosis of major depression in adulthood: A controlled study.* Journal of Affective Disorders, 112(1-3), 112-119. doi: 10.1016/j.jad.2008.04.015

14. O'Rourke, T. W., Ellis, T. E., & Clark, M. A. (2016). *Somatic symptom disorder: An overview of assessment, treatment, and cultural factors.* American Family Physician, 94(9), 731-738.

15. Pearsall, P. *The Heart's Code: Tapping the Wisdom and Power of Our Heart Energy,* Harmony; Reprint edition (April 6, 1999)

16. Pearsall, P.; Schwartz, G. E.; Russek, L. G. *"Organ Transplants and Cellular Memories"* Extracted from Nexus Magazine, Volume 12, Number 3 (April - May 2005)

17. Scarpa, A. *Tabulae neurologicae: Ad illustrandam historiam anatomicam: Cardiacorum nervorum, noni nervorum cerebri, glossopharyngaei, et pharyngaei ex octavo cerebri.* Apud Balthassarem Comini. **1794.** [**Google Scholar**]

18. Smith, T. W., Cribbet, M. R., Nealey-Moore, J. B., Uchino, B. N., Williams, P. G., MacKenzie, J., & Thayer, J. F. (2011). *Matters of the variable heart: Respiratory sinus arrhythmia response to marital interaction and associations with marital quality.* Journal of Personality and Social Psychology, 100(1), 103 –119. https://doi.org/10.1037/a0021136

19. **Swan, T. (2016). *The Completion Process. The Practice of putting yourself back together again.* Hay House Publishing**

20. Swan, T. (2018). *The anatomy of loneliness. How to find your way back to connection.* Penguin Random House

21. Swan, T. (2023) https://www.youtube.com/@TealSwanOfficial

22. Swan, T. (2023) tealswan.com/premium/workshops

23. Thayer, J. F., Yamamoto, S. S., & Brosschot, J. F. (2010). *The relationship of autonomic imbalance, heart rate variability and cardiovascular disease risk factors.* International journal of cardiology, 141(2), 122-131.

24. Tops, M., & Boksem, M. A. (2011). *Emotional regulation, interpersonal dominance, and resting frontal asymmetry: A study with EEG and ECG.* Biological psychology, 87(1), 106-112.

25. Vining, E., et al. (1997). *Why would you remove half a brain? The outcome of 58 children after hemispherectomy-the Johns Hopkins experience: 1968 to 1996.* Pediatrics 1997 Aug 100(2 Pt 1):163-71. doi: 10.1542/peds.100.2.163. https://pubmed.ncbi.nlm.nih.gov/9240794/

www.emotionaltraumaclinics.com

About Us

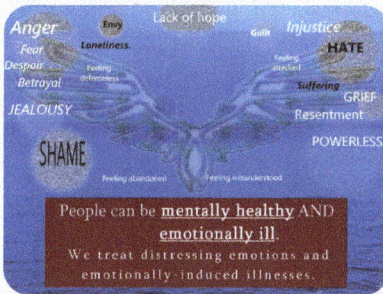

Welcome to our revolutionary Clinic for Emotions, the first of its kind in the world!

Here, we provide a safe and nurturing space for you to heal your emotional wounds and improve your overall emotional, mental and physical well-being.

Unlike traditional mental health establishments, we focus on emotions and their coping mechanisms, eliminating any diagnosis or stigma associated with mental health.

Our multi-layered emotional integration therapy is tailored specifically to address your individual emotional wounds, allowing you to experience true healing and personal growth- and a much better quality of life.

Trust our team of dedicated professionals to guide you through this transformative journey towards emotional balance and inner peace. Your emotional well-being is our priority, and we are here to support you every step of the way.

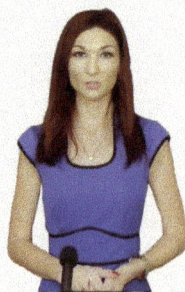

Emotional Trauma Clinics
Transforming pain into peace

Home   Services   Shop   Circle of Friends   Contact   Join our team

BOOK NOW

We are here for you because we care.

Our therapists offer, first and foremost, emotional presence- a warm heart. You will not be talking to a cold face.

How are you feeling today?

We can help you with:

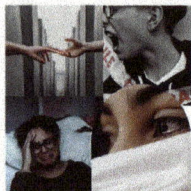

Distressing feelings/ emotions

- Loneliness
- Fear/Anxiety
- Despair
- Shame
- Hopelessness
- Grief
- Resentment
- Guilt
- Injustice
- Anger/Rage
- Envy
- Jealousy
- Feeling abandoned
- Feeling attacked
- Feeling unseen

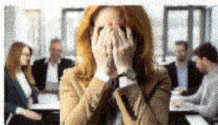

Traumatising life experiences

- Victim of bullying
- Physical, emotional or mental abuse
- Sexual abuse
- Social rejection
- Being humiliated
- Being wrongfully accused/ scapegoated
- Inability to leave an abusive relationship
- Other life experiences that cause painful emotional reactions

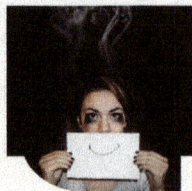

Dysfunctional coping mechanisms

- Suicide ideation or attempts
- Substance use -alcohol, nicotine, other stimulants (opioids, sedatives, etc)
- Gambling
- Over-eating
- Over-fasting
- Inappropriate sexual arousal
- Dissociation/multiple personalities
- any repeated behaviours that have negative life consequences